HBOT HEALING HORIZONS

A Holistic Approach to Healing Numerous Health Conditions with Hyperbaric Oxygen Therapeutic Potential

Dr Zoe Zurich

INTRODUCTION

Understanding Hyperbaric Oxygen Therapy

Hyperbaric Oxygen Therapy (HBOT) stands at the intersection of medical science and engineering, offering a promising avenue for healing and recovery across a wide spectrum of health conditions. At its core, HBOT involves the administration of pure oxygen at increased atmospheric pressure within a specially designed chamber. This therapeutic approach capitalizes on the physiological effects of oxygen under pressure to enhance tissue oxygenation, promote wound healing, reduce inflammation, and stimulate various cellular processes vital for recovery.

History and Evolution

The roots of hyperbaric therapy trace back to the mid-1600s when pioneering experiments by English physician and clergyman, Henshaw, explored the effects of pressurized air on health. However, it wasn't until the 20th century that hyperbaric medicine began to take shape with the development of pressurized chambers for diving and subsequent observations of their therapeutic benefits. In the 1930s, researchers recognized the potential of hyperbaric oxygen in treating decompression sickness, laying the groundwork for its medical application.

Principles of Hyperbaric Oxygen Therapy

Central to understanding HBOT is grasping its underlying principles. The therapy operates on the premise that increasing atmospheric pressure allows greater dissolution of oxygen in bodily fluids, including plasma, cerebrospinal fluid, and interstitial fluid. This heightened oxygen availability drives a range of physiological responses, such as vasoconstriction and increased oxygen delivery to tissues, leading to improved oxygenation of hypoxic areas. Moreover, HBOT promotes the formation of reactive oxygen species (ROS) which play a crucial role in antimicrobial activity, angiogenesis, and tissue repair.

Mechanisms of Action

HBOT exerts its therapeutic effects through multifaceted mechanisms involving both oxygen-dependent and oxygen-independent pathways. Oxygen under pressure enhances oxygen transport capacity, facilitating oxygen diffusion to tissues with compromised blood flow. Additionally, HBOT mitigates ischemia-reperfusion injury by reducing oxidative stress and inflammation, preserving tissue viability following episodes of vascular compromise. Furthermore, HBOT modulates immune responses, augmenting phagocytic activity and cytokine production to combat infection and promote tissue regeneration.

Clinical Applications

The versatility of HBOT extends across a diverse array of medical conditions, encompassing acute and chronic ailments alike. In wound care, HBOT serves as a potent adjunctive therapy for refractory ulcers, diabetic foot wounds, and radiation-induced tissue damage, fostering granulation tissue formation and accelerating wound closure. Neurological disorders, including stroke, traumatic brain injury, and cerebral palsy, benefit from HBOT's neuroprotective and neuroregenerative properties, promoting functional recovery and mitigating secondary brain injury. Additionally, HBOT finds utility in treating carbon monoxide poisoning, enhancing oxygenation and displacing toxic carbon monoxide from hemoglobin, thereby preventing cellular hypoxia and mitigating neurological sequelae.

In essence, understanding hyperbaric oxygen therapy requires delving into its historical roots, elucidating its fundamental principles, elucidating its mechanisms of action, and surveying its diverse clinical applications. As research continues to unravel the intricacies of HBOT, its role in modern medicine is poised to expand, offering new avenues for healing and restoration across a broad spectrum of health conditions

In crafting a book on Hyperbaric Oxygen Therapy (HBOT), it's essential to delineate its purpose and the scope it aims to cover. This section serves as a guiding beacon, outlining the overarching goals of the book and the breadth of topics it endeavors to explore. From elucidating the therapeutic potential of HBOT to providing practical insights into its clinical applications, the purpose and scope of the book set the stage for an insightful and comprehensive exploration of this fascinating therapeutic modality.

At the heart of this book lies a quest to demystify Hyperbaric Oxygen Therapy and unravel its therapeutic intricacies. Readers will embark on a journey of discovery, delving into the historical roots, fundamental principles, and mechanisms of action that underpin this innovative treatment approach. By elucidating the science behind HBOT, the book aims to empower readers with a deeper understanding of how oxygen under pressure exerts its healing effects, paving the way for informed decision-making and clinical practice.

A core facet of the book's scope revolves around exploring the diverse array of clinical applications for HBOT and distilling the wealth of evidence supporting its efficacy. From wound healing and neurological disorders to carbon monoxide poisoning and radiation injury, HBOT boasts a broad spectrum of therapeutic indications, each grounded in rigorous scientific inquiry. Through an evidence-based lens, the book seeks to provide clinicians, researchers, and patients alike with a comprehensive overview of the indications, protocols, and outcomes associated with HBOT across various medical conditions.

Patient Education and Empowerment

Central to the ethos of this book is the mission to empower patients with knowledge and agency in their healthcare journey. By offering insights into the patient experience, testimonials of healing and recovery, and practical guidance on navigating HBOT treatment, the book aims to serve as a beacon of hope and information for individuals grappling with health challenges. Through clear, accessible language and relatable anecdotes, readers will find solace, inspiration, and actionable advice to navigate the complexities of HBOT with confidence and resilience.

Practical Considerations and Implementation

Beyond theoretical discourse, the book endeavors to equip healthcare professionals with practical tools and insights to integrate HBOT into clinical practice effectively. From patient selection and treatment planning to chamber operation and safety protocols, readers will gain actionable strategies and best practices to optimize the delivery of HBOT in diverse healthcare settings. By addressing logistical considerations, regulatory guidelines, and interdisciplinary collaboration, the book aims to foster a culture of excellence and safety in the provision of HBOT services worldwide.

Future Directions and Innovation

As the landscape of healthcare continues to evolve, so too does the frontier of Hyperbaric Oxygen Therapy. In charting the future trajectory of HBOT, the book explores emerging trends, technological advancements, and novel applications poised to shape the field in the years to come. By embracing innovation and fostering dialogue among researchers, clinicians, and industry stakeholders, the book aspires to catalyze progress and innovation in HBOT, unlocking new frontiers of healing and discovery.

In essence, the purpose and scope of this book are multifaceted, encompassing education, empowerment, and innovation in the realm of Hyperbaric Oxygen Therapy. By illuminating the science, clinical applications, and future horizons of HBOT, the book aims to inspire readers, foster dialogue, and advance the collective understanding of this transformative therapeutic modality. Whether you're a healthcare professional seeking to expand your clinical toolkit, a patient embarking on a healing journey, or a curious mind eager to explore the frontiers of medical science, this book invites you to embark on a voyage of discovery and healing through the power of oxygen under pressure.

CHAPTER 1

FOUNDATIONS OF HYPERBARIC OXYGEN THERAPY

Hyperbaric Oxygen Therapy (HBOT) stands as a testament to the intricate interplay between medical science, engineering, and human physiology. In this foundational chapter, we embark on a journey to explore the historical origins, fundamental principles, and mechanistic underpinnings that define HBOT as a cornerstone of modern medicine. From its humble beginnings as a tool for deep-sea divers to its evolution into a potent therapeutic modality with diverse clinical applications, HBOT epitomizes the marriage of scientific curiosity and clinical innovation.

Historical Origins

The roots of hyperbaric therapy trace back centuries, intertwining with the rich tapestry of exploration, discovery, and scientific inquiry. In the 17th century, pioneering experiments by English clergyman and polymath, Henshaw, laid the groundwork for our understanding of pressurized air and its effects on human health. However, it wasn't until the 20th century that hyperbaric medicine began to take shape, propelled by advancements in diving technology and the serendipitous observations of its therapeutic benefits. From the treatment of decompression sickness in divers to the management of carbon monoxide poisoning and wound healing, the historical trajectory of HBOT is marked by a series of landmark discoveries and paradigm shifts that continue to shape its clinical practice today.

Fundamental Principles

At its core, HBOT operates on the principle that exposing the body to increased atmospheric pressure enhances the delivery and dissolution of oxygen in bodily fluids, thereby augmenting tissue oxygenation and promoting healing. This fundamental premise rests on the laws of physics and gas behavior, wherein Boyle's Law dictates that the volume of a gas decreases with increasing pressure, leading to greater oxygen solubility in blood and tissues. Moreover, Henry's Law underscores the principle of gas diffusion, wherein the partial pressure of a gas determines its concentration in solution, further elucidating the mechanisms by which oxygen exerts its therapeutic effects under hyperbaric conditions.

Mechanistic Underpinnings

Delving deeper into the mechanistic underpinnings of HBOT unveils a complex interplay of physiological responses and cellular pathways that drive therapeutic outcomes. Under hyperbaric conditions, oxygen diffuses across biological membranes and enters tissues with compromised blood flow, providing a vital oxygen reserve to fuel cellular metabolism and mitigate hypoxic injury. Moreover, HBOT promotes the generation of reactive oxygen species (ROS), which serve as signaling molecules to modulate immune responses, stimulate angiogenesis, and enhance tissue repair mechanisms. By harnessing the dual effects of increased oxygen delivery and ROS-mediated signaling, HBOT exerts a myriad of beneficial effects across a spectrum of acute and chronic medical conditions, from wound healing and neurological disorders to infectious diseases and radiation injury.

Clinical Considerations

In translating these foundational principles into clinical practice, several key considerations come to the fore, including patient selection, treatment protocols, and safety precautions. Patient evaluation and assessment play a crucial role in determining the suitability of HBOT and tailoring treatment plans to individual needs and medical conditions. Standard treatment protocols, encompassing varying pressures, durations, and frequencies, provide a framework for delivering HBOT across different clinical scenarios, while adherence to safety guidelines and regulatory standards ensures the welfare of patients and healthcare providers alike.

In summary, this lays the groundwork for our exploration of Hyperbaric Oxygen Therapy, tracing its historical origins, elucidating its fundamental principles, and unraveling the mechanistic underpinnings that underlie its therapeutic efficacy. As we delve deeper into the realm of HBOT, we invite readers to embark on a journey of discovery and inquiry, as we seek to unlock the mysteries of oxygen under pressure and harness its healing potential for the betterment of human health and well-being.

CHAPTER 2

History and Evolution of Hyperbaric Oxygen Therapy

The history and evolution of Hyperbaric Oxygen Therapy (HBOT) are deeply intertwined with humanity's quest for exploration, discovery, and the conquest of new frontiers. From its humble origins in ancient civilizations to its modern-day applications in cutting-edge medicine, the journey of HBOT is a testament to human ingenuity, resilience, and the relentless pursuit of knowledge.

Ancient Origins

While the formalization of hyperbaric therapy as a medical intervention emerged in the 20th century, traces of its usage can be found in ancient civilizations dating back thousands of years. Historical accounts from civilizations such as the Greeks, Egyptians, and Chinese document the use of pressurized environments for therapeutic purposes, albeit with rudimentary understanding and crude implementations. From submerging patients in water-filled vessels to early attempts at creating pressurized chambers, these ancient practices laid the groundwork for the eventual development of modern hyperbaric medicine.

Early Experiments and Discoveries

The dawn of modern hyperbaric medicine can be traced to the 17th century, when pioneering experiments by English polymath, Henshaw, shed light on the physiological effects of pressurized air on human health. Henshaw's "Domicilium" or "Diving Bell" served as a precursor to the hyperbaric chamber, allowing individuals to descend to greater depths underwater while experiencing increased atmospheric pressure. These early experiments paved the way for subsequent discoveries in the realm of diving medicine and laid the foundation for the development of hyperbaric oxygen therapy.

Emergence as a Medical Intervention

The 20th century witnessed a paradigm shift in the perception and application of hyperbaric therapy, spurred by advancements in diving technology and the burgeoning field of aviation medicine. In the 1930s, researchers such as Behnke and Shaw recognized the therapeutic potential of hyperbaric oxygen in treating decompression sickness, a condition afflicting divers subjected to rapid changes in pressure. Subsequent studies elucidated the benefits of HBOT in enhancing tissue oxygenation, promoting wound healing, and mitigating the effects of carbon monoxide poisoning, further solidifying its role as a legitimate medical intervention.

Clinical Applications and Milestones

The clinical applications of HBOT expanded exponentially throughout the 20th century, driven by a growing body of scientific evidence and technological innovations in hyperbaric chamber design. Milestones such as the establishment of the Undersea and Hyperbaric Medical Society (UHMS) in 1967 and the publication of seminal works like "Hyperbaric Oxygen Therapy:

A Committee Report" in 1977, served to standardize treatment protocols and foster collaboration among researchers and clinicians in the field. Over the ensuing decades, HBOT gained recognition as a valuable adjunctive therapy for conditions ranging from diabetic foot ulcers and radiation injury to traumatic brain injury and neurologic disorders, solidifying its position as a cornerstone of modern medicine.

Technological Advancements and Future Directions

The 21st century has witnessed a proliferation of technological advancements in hyperbaric chamber design, ranging from monoplace chambers for single-patient use to multiplace chambers capable of accommodating medical teams and equipment. Innovations such as hyperbaric oxygen tents and portable chambers have expanded the accessibility of HBOT beyond traditional hospital settings, enabling treatment in remote locations and emergency situations. Moreover, ongoing research endeavors continue to explore novel applications of HBOT in areas such as regenerative medicine, neurorehabilitation, and immunotherapy, paving the way for exciting breakthroughs and discoveries in the years to come.

In conclusion, the history and evolution of Hyperbaric Oxygen Therapy are a testament to human curiosity, perseverance, and the relentless pursuit of scientific inquiry. From ancient civilizations to modern medical practice, the journey of HBOT embodies the spirit of exploration and innovation, offering new hope and healing to generations past, present, and future. As we stand on the cusp of a new era of discovery, the legacy of HBOT serves as a beacon of inspiration, guiding us towards a future where the frontiers of medicine continue to expand, and the boundaries of human potential are continually pushed to new heights.

Hyperbaric Oxygen Therapy (HBOT) operates on a set of fundamental principles rooted in physics, physiology, and clinical medicine. Understanding these principles is essential for grasping how HBOT exerts its therapeutic effects and optimizing its application in clinical practice. In this section, we delve into the core principles that underpin HBOT, ranging from gas laws to oxygen transport mechanisms, providing a comprehensive framework for its implementation and interpretation.

Gas Laws and Pressure

At the heart of HBOT lies the principle of gas laws, which govern the behavior of gases under different pressure conditions. Boyle's Law states that the volume of a gas is inversely proportional to its pressure, meaning that as pressure increases, the volume of a gas decreases. This principle is critical in hyperbaric chambers, where increased atmospheric pressure leads to greater oxygen solubility in bodily fluids and tissues. Additionally, Henry's Law dictates that the amount of gas dissolved in a liquid is directly proportional to its partial pressure, further elucidating how HBOT enhances oxygen delivery to tissues.

Oxygen Transport and Delivery

HBOT enhances oxygen transport and delivery through several mechanisms, capitalizing on the increased oxygen solubility in blood and tissues under hyperbaric conditions. By elevating atmospheric pressure, HBOT increases the partial pressure of oxygen in inspired air, leading to a greater concentration of dissolved oxygen in plasma and facilitating oxygen diffusion to tissues with compromised blood flow. Moreover, HBOT promotes the formation of oxygen-rich microbubbles in plasma, which can reach areas of tissue ischemia and augment oxygen delivery, even in regions with impaired blood flow.

Physiological Responses

Under hyperbaric conditions, the body undergoes a series of physiological responses that contribute to the therapeutic effects of HBOT.

Vasoconstriction occurs in response to increased atmospheric pressure, redistributing blood flow to vital organs and tissues and optimizing oxygen delivery. Oxygen diffusion gradients drive the penetration of oxygen into ischemic tissues, alleviating hypoxia and promoting cellular metabolism and energy production. Furthermore, HBOT stimulates the release of growth factors and cytokines, which play a crucial role in tissue repair, angiogenesis, and immune modulation, fostering a regenerative microenvironment conducive to healing.

Clinical Applications

The principles of HBOT find application across a diverse array of medical conditions, spanning acute injuries, chronic diseases, and emergent indications. In wound healing, HBOT promotes angiogenesis and collagen synthesis, accelerates epithelialization, and enhances the bactericidal activity of leukocytes, facilitating the resolution of infections and promoting tissue repair. Neurological disorders benefit from HBOT's neuroprotective and neuroregenerative effects, which include reducing cerebral edema, improving oxygenation of ischemic brain tissue, and promoting synaptic plasticity and neuronal recovery.

Safety and Monitoring

While HBOT offers a wealth of therapeutic benefits, it is essential to adhere to safety guidelines and monitor patients closely to mitigate potential risks and complications. Barotrauma, oxygen toxicity, and claustrophobia are among the most common adverse effects associated with HBOT, necessitating vigilant monitoring and appropriate interventions. Patient selection, pre-treatment evaluations, and adherence to established treatment protocols are crucial in ensuring the safety and efficacy of HBOT, minimizing the risk of adverse events and optimizing patient outcomes.

In summary, the principles of Hyperbaric Oxygen Therapy encompass a nuanced understanding of gas laws, oxygen transport mechanisms, physiological responses, and clinical applications. By leveraging the principles of HBOT, clinicians can harness the therapeutic potential of oxygen under pressure to promote healing, alleviate suffering, and improve quality of life for patients across a broad spectrum of medical conditions. As our understanding of HBOT continues to evolve, so too will our ability to unlock new frontiers of healing and discovery, ushering in a future where the promise of oxygen under pressure is realized in its fullest capacity.

Hyperbaric Oxygen Therapy (HBOT) exerts its therapeutic effects through a complex interplay of physiological responses and cellular mechanisms, spanning from the molecular level to the systemic level. In this section, we delve into the intricate mechanisms by which HBOT promotes healing, mitigates injury, and enhances physiological function, shedding light on the diverse pathways through which oxygen under pressure exerts its beneficial effects.

Oxygen Transport and Diffusion

Central to the mechanism of action of HBOT is the enhanced transport and diffusion of oxygen in bodily fluids and tissues under hyperbaric conditions. By increasing atmospheric pressure, HBOT elevates the partial pressure of oxygen in inspired air, leading to greater oxygen solubility in plasma and tissues. This heightened oxygen availability drives oxygen diffusion gradients, enabling oxygen to penetrate ischemic tissues, bypassing compromised blood flow and delivering vital oxygen to hypoxic cells.

Oxygenation of Ischemic Tissues

One of the primary therapeutic effects of HBOT is the oxygenation of ischemic tissues, where compromised blood flow results in inadequate oxygen delivery and cellular hypoxia. Under hyperbaric conditions, oxygen diffuses across biological membranes and enters tissues with impaired perfusion, restoring oxygen tension and promoting cellular metabolism and energy production. This oxygen-mediated rescue of ischemic tissues plays a pivotal role in mitigating tissue damage, preventing cell death, and fostering tissue repair and regeneration.

Anti-inflammatory and Anti-edema Effects

HBOT exerts potent anti-inflammatory and anti-edema effects, which are particularly relevant in the context of acute injuries and inflammatory conditions. By reducing inflammation and edema, HBOT helps alleviate tissue pressure, improve microcirculation, and enhance oxygen delivery to affected areas. Moreover, HBOT modulates the release of inflammatory mediators and cytokines, dampening the inflammatory response and promoting resolution of tissue injury, thereby facilitating the healing process and mitigating secondary tissue damage.

Stimulation of Angiogenesis and Tissue Repair

Angiogenesis, the formation of new blood vessels from pre-existing vasculature, is a critical component of tissue repair and regeneration. HBOT promotes angiogenesis through various mechanisms, including upregulation of vascular endothelial growth factor (VEGF), stimulation of endothelial cell proliferation and migration, and enhancement of pericyte recruitment and vessel maturation. This neovascularization facilitates the delivery of oxygen and nutrients to healing tissues, accelerates wound closure, and promotes tissue remodeling and scar formation.

Antimicrobial Activity

HBOT exhibits broad-spectrum antimicrobial activity against a wide range of pathogens, including bacteria, viruses, fungi, and protozoa. The bactericidal and bacteriostatic effects of HBOT are attributed to several mechanisms, including direct oxidative damage to microbial membranes, inhibition of microbial metabolism, and modulation of host immune responses. Moreover, HBOT enhances the activity of leukocytes and macrophages, potentiating the innate immune response and augmenting microbial clearance, making it a valuable adjunctive therapy in the management of infections and wound healing.

Neuroprotective and Neuroregenerative Effects

In the realm of neurology, HBOT demonstrates neuroprotective and neuroregenerative properties, offering promise for the treatment of traumatic brain injury, stroke, neurodegenerative diseases, and other neurological disorders. HBOT mitigates neuronal injury by reducing cerebral edema, suppressing neuroinflammation, and preserving mitochondrial function. Furthermore, HBOT promotes neuroplasticity and synaptic remodeling, facilitating functional recovery and neuronal regeneration in the injured or diseased brain.

In conclusion, the mechanisms of action of Hyperbaric Oxygen Therapy are multifaceted, encompassing oxygen transportand diffusion, oxygenation of ischemic tissues, anti-inflammatory and anti-edema effects, stimulation of angiogenesis and tissue repair, antimicrobial activity, and neuroprotective/neuroregenerative effects. By leveraging these diverse mechanisms, HBOT exerts a profound influence on cellular physiology, tissue function, and systemic homeostasis, fostering an environment conducive to healing, regeneration, and recovery.

Enhanced Cellular Metabolism

Under hyperbaric conditions, oxygen acts as a substrate for cellular metabolism, fueling biochemical reactions essential for cellular function and viability. By elevating tissue oxygen tension, HBOT enhances aerobic metabolism, ATP production, and oxidative phosphorylation, providing cells with the energy required for cellular repair, proliferation, and maintenance. This metabolic boost is particularly crucial in tissues undergoing repair or regeneration, where increased energy demands must be met to support the healing process.

Modulation of Oxidative Stress

While oxygen is indispensable for cellular metabolism and energy production, it can also give rise to reactive oxygen species (ROS) through incomplete reduction of molecular oxygen. Under normal physiological conditions, ROS play a dual role as signaling molecules and mediators of oxidative stress, contributing to cellular homeostasis and defense mechanisms. However, excessive ROS production can overwhelm endogenous antioxidant defenses, leading to oxidative damage, inflammation, and tissue injury. HBOT modulates oxidative stress by enhancing ROS scavenging capacity, upregulating antioxidant enzyme activity, and restoring redox balance, thereby mitigating cellular damage and promoting tissue resilience.

Immune Modulation

HBOT exerts profound effects on the immune system, modulating immune cell function, cytokine production, and inflammatory responses. By enhancing oxygen delivery to immune cells and inflamed tissues, HBOT boosts immune surveillance and potentiates antimicrobial activity, aiding in the clearance of pathogens and promoting resolution of infections. Moreover, HBOT modulates the release of pro-inflammatory and anti-inflammatory cytokines, shifting the balance towards a more anti-inflammatory phenotype, which is conducive to tissue repair and resolution of inflammation.

Neuroplasticity and Cognitive Function

In the realm of neuroscience, HBOT holds promise for enhancing neuroplasticity, cognitive function, and neurological recovery following injury or disease. HBOT stimulates neurogenesis, synaptogenesis, and dendritic branching, facilitating synaptic remodeling and functional recovery in the injured or diseased brain. Moreover, HBOT enhances cerebral blood flow, oxygenation, and glucose metabolism, providing the energy substrates required for neuronal repair and regeneration. These neuroregenerative effects underpin HBOT's potential for treating neurodegenerative diseases, traumatic brain injury, and other neurological disorders, offering new hope for patients with limited treatment options.

In summary, the mechanisms of action of Hyperbaric Oxygen Therapy are vast and multifaceted, encompassing a myriad of cellular, molecular, and systemic responses. By harnessing the power of oxygen under pressure, HBOT exerts a profound influence on tissue physiology, immune function, neuroplasticity, and cellular metabolism, offering new avenues for healing, regeneration, and recovery. As our understanding of HBOT continues to evolve, so too will our ability to unlock its full therapeutic potential, ushering in a new era of personalized medicine and transformative healthcare interventions.

CHAPTER 3:

Medical Conditions and Applications

Now we embark on a comprehensive exploration of the diverse array of medical conditions and applications for Hyperbaric Oxygen Therapy (HBOT). From acute injuries to chronic diseases, HBOT has emerged as a versatile therapeutic modality with broad-ranging clinical utility. By delving into the evidence-based indications, treatment protocols, and outcomes associated with HBOT across various medical domains, this chapter aims to provide clinicians, researchers, and patients alike with a comprehensive understanding of its therapeutic potential and application in modern healthcare.

Wound Healing and Tissue Repair

One of the most well-established applications of HBOT lies in the realm of wound healing and tissue repair. HBOT promotes angiogenesis, collagen synthesis, and fibroblast proliferation, accelerating the formation of granulation tissue and facilitating wound closure. In diabetic foot ulcers, HBOT enhances oxygen delivery to ischemic tissues, promotes neovascularization, and mitigates infection, leading to improved healing rates and reduced amputation risk. Similarly, HBOT is effective in treating chronic wounds, pressure ulcers, and non-healing surgical incisions, offering new hope for patients with recalcitrant wounds that fail to respond to conventional therapies.

Carbon Monoxide Poisoning and Toxic Gas Exposure

HBOT serves as a lifesaving intervention in the management of carbon monoxide poisoning and toxic gas exposure. Carbon monoxide (CO) has a high affinity for hemoglobin, displacing oxygen and leading to tissue hypoxia and cellular injury. HBOT facilitates the elimination of CO from hemoglobin, enhances tissue oxygenation, and accelerates the clearance of CO from the bloodstream. Moreover, HBOT mitigates oxidative stress, reduces inflammatory responses, and promotes neuronal recovery, minimizing the risk of long-term neurological sequelae and improving clinical outcomes in patients with acute CO poisoning.

Radiation Injury and Late Radiation Effects

In the realm of oncology, HBOT holds promise for mitigating the adverse effects of radiation therapy and enhancing tissue recovery following radiation injury. Radiation therapy is a cornerstone of cancer treatment, but it can cause collateral damage to surrounding healthy tissues, leading to radiation-induced tissue injury and late radiation effects. HBOT mitigates radiation-induced fibrosis, promotes tissue reoxygenation, and enhances the repair of damaged DNA, mitigating the risk of late radiation effects such as soft tissue necrosis, osteoradionecrosis, and radiation cystitis. Additionally, HBOT may potentiate the efficacy of radiation therapy by overcoming tumor hypoxia and enhancing radiosensitivity, offering new avenues for combination therapy in oncology.

Neurological Disorders and Traumatic Brain Injury

Neurological disorders represent another frontier in the application of HBOT, with promising results emerging in conditions such as traumatic brain injury (TBI), stroke, and neurodegenerative diseases. In TBI, HBOT reduces cerebral edema, improves cerebral blood flow, and enhances neuronal survival and synaptic plasticity, leading to improved neurological outcomes and functional recovery. Similarly, in acute ischemic stroke, HBOT promotes reperfusion, reduces infarct size, and enhances neurogenesis and angiogenesis, offering new hope for patients with limited treatment options. Moreover, HBOT shows potential for slowing disease progression and improving cognitive function in neurodegenerative diseases such as Alzheimer's disease and

Parkinson's disease, although further research is needed to elucidate its long-term efficacy and safety in these populations.

Infectious Diseases and Immunomodulation

HBOT exhibits broad-spectrum antimicrobial activity and immunomodulatory effects, making it a valuable adjunctive therapy in the management of infectious diseases and immune-mediated disorders. HBOT enhances oxygen-dependent antimicrobial mechanisms, such as oxidative killing by leukocytes and inhibition of microbial metabolism, thereby augmenting the host immune response and promoting microbial clearance. In conditions such as necrotizing soft tissue infections, osteomyelitis, and refractory infections,

HBOT complements conventional antimicrobial therapy, accelerates wound healing, and reduces the risk of complications such as amputation and sepsis. Moreover, HBOT modulates inflammatory responses, suppresses cytokine production, and promotes the resolution of inflammation, offering new avenues for the treatment of immune-mediated disorders such as inflammatory bowel disease, rheumatoid arthritis, and autoimmune encephalitis.

Other Emerging Applications

Beyond the established indications, HBOT is being explored for a myriad of emerging applications, ranging from sports medicine and aesthetic procedures to regenerative medicine and anti-aging interventions. In sports medicine, HBOT accelerates recovery from musculoskeletal injuries, reduces inflammation, and enhances tissue repair, allowing athletes to return to play more quickly and with reduced risk of complications. In aesthetic procedures, HBOT promotes collagen synthesis, accelerates wound healing, and enhances skin rejuvenation, offering new avenues for non-invasive cosmetic enhancement. Moreover, in regenerative medicine, HBOT stimulates stem cell mobilization and differentiation, enhances tissue regeneration, and promotes organ repair, holding promise for the treatment of conditions such as myocardial infarction, peripheral artery disease, and spinal cord injury. Additionally, in the realm of anti-aging medicine, HBOT combats oxidative stress, promotes cellular repair mechanisms, and enhances mitochondrial function, offering new strategies for slowing the aging process and improving overall health and longevity.

In conclusion, this provides a comprehensive overview of the diverse array of medical conditions and applications for Hyperbaric Oxygen Therapy. From wound healing and tissue repair to neurological disorders, infectious diseases, and emerging indications, HBOT offers new avenues for healing, recovery, and regeneration across a broad spectrum of medical specialties. By elucidating the evidence-based indications, treatment protocols, and outcomes associated with HBOT, this chapter aims to empower clinicians, researchers, and patients alike with the knowledge and tools needed to harness the full therapeutic potential of oxygen under pressure in modern healthcare.

Hyperbaric Oxygen Therapy (HBOT) has emerged as a valuable adjunctive treatment modality for promoting the healing of wounds and injuries across a diverse spectrum of medical conditions. By harnessing the therapeutic effects of oxygen under increased atmospheric pressure, HBOT enhances tissue oxygenation, promotes angiogenesis, reduces inflammation, and accelerates wound closure, offering new hope for patients with chronic or non-healing wounds.

Mechanisms of Action

The mechanisms by which HBOT promotes wound healing are multifaceted and involve a complex interplay of physiological responses at the cellular and molecular levels. Under hyperbaric conditions, oxygen diffuses into ischemic tissues, bypassing compromised blood flow and delivering oxygen to hypoxic cells, thereby promoting cellular metabolism and energy production. Moreover, HBOT stimulates the release of growth factors, such as vascular endothelial growth factor (VEGF) and fibroblast growth factor (FGF), which promote angiogenesis, collagen synthesis, and fibroblast proliferation, facilitating the formation of granulation tissue and wound closure. Additionally, HBOT enhances the bactericidal activity of leukocytes, inhibits microbial growth, and promotes tissue oxygenation, thereby reducing the risk of infection and promoting a sterile wound environment conducive to healing.

HBOT finds application in a wide range of wound types, including diabetic foot ulcers, venous ulcers, pressure ulcers, non-healing surgical wounds, and traumatic injuries. In diabetic foot ulcers, HBOT improves tissue oxygenation, promotes angiogenesis, and accelerates wound healing rates, reducing the risk of infection and amputation. Similarly, in venous ulcers, HBOT enhances tissue perfusion, reduces edema, and promotes collagen synthesis, leading to improved wound healing outcomes and reduced recurrence rates. Moreover, HBOT is effective in treating pressure ulcers, where it promotes tissue oxygenation, reduces inflammation, and facilitates the resolution of infections, thereby accelerating wound closure and preventing complications such as sepsis and osteomyelitis. Additionally, in non-healing surgical wounds and traumatic injuries, HBOT enhances tissue repair mechanisms, reduces wound complications, and improves overall healing rates, offering new avenues for surgical and trauma patients with complex wound care needs.

Evidence-Based Practice

The efficacy of HBOT in wound healing is supported by a growing body of clinical evidence, including randomized controlled trials, meta-analyses, and systematic reviews. Numerous studies have demonstrated the beneficial effects of HBOT in promoting wound healing, reducing healing time, and improving clinical outcomes across various wound types and patient populations. Meta-analyses have shown that HBOT significantly increases the likelihood of wound healing and reduces the risk of major amputations in patients with diabetic foot ulcers. Moreover, systematic reviews have reported consistent improvements in wound healing rates, infection control, and quality of life outcomes in patients receiving HBOT for chronic or non-healing wounds. These findings underscore the importance of incorporating HBOT into the multidisciplinary management of complex wounds, where conventional therapies have proven ineffective or insufficient.

Hyperbaric Oxygen Therapy holds promise as a valuable adjunctive treatment modality for promoting the healing of wounds and injuries across a diverse spectrum of medical conditions. By leveraging the therapeutic effects of oxygen under increased atmospheric pressure, HBOT enhances tissue oxygenation, promotes angiogenesis, reduces inflammation, and accelerates wound closure, offering new avenues for patients with chronic or non-healing wounds. As our understanding of the mechanisms underlying HBOT continues to evolve, so too will our ability to optimize its application and maximize its therapeutic benefits in wound care and tissue repair.

Alleviating Chronic Fatigue Syndrome

Chronic Fatigue Syndrome (CFS), also known as myalgic encephalomyelitis (ME), is a complex and debilitating condition characterized by persistent fatigue, cognitive dysfunction, and other symptoms that significantly impair daily functioning and quality of life. While the etiology of CFS remains poorly understood, emerging evidence suggests that Hyperbaric Oxygen Therapy (HBOT) may offer therapeutic benefits in alleviating symptoms and improving overall well-being for individuals with this challenging condition.

Symptoms and Impact of Chronic Fatigue Syndrome

CFS presents with a constellation of symptoms that extend beyond mere fatigue, encompassing cognitive impairment, unrefreshing sleep, post-exertional malaise, and autonomic dysfunction. These symptoms are often chronic and debilitating, leading to profound physical, cognitive, and emotional impairment, as well as significant social and occupational dysfunction. The exact cause of CFS remains elusive, with theories implicating immune dysfunction, neuroinflammation, mitochondrial dysfunction, and dysregulation of the autonomic nervous system. Despite decades of research, effective treatments for CFS remain limited, leaving patients and healthcare providers alike searching for novel therapeutic interventions to alleviate symptoms and improve quality of life.

Therapeutic Potential of HBOT

HBOT holds promise as a potential therapeutic intervention for individuals with CFS due to its ability to enhance tissue oxygenation, promote mitochondrial function, and modulate inflammatory responses. Under hyperbaric conditions, oxygen is dissolved in plasma at supraphysiological levels, bypassing compromised blood flow and delivering oxygen to hypoxic tissues. This oxygen-rich environment promotes cellular metabolism, ATP production, and mitochondrial biogenesis, addressing the underlying energy deficits and oxidative stress associated with CFS. Moreover, HBOT modulates inflammatory cytokines, such as interleukin-6 (IL-6) and tumor necrosis factor-alpha (TNF-α), reducing neuroinflammation and mitigating symptoms such as cognitive dysfunction and post-exertional malaise.

Clinical Evidence and Outcomes

While clinical research on the use of HBOT in CFS is still in its infancy, preliminary studies and case reports have shown promising results in improving symptoms and functional outcomes for individuals with this condition. A small pilot study conducted by Rowe et al. (2015) demonstrated that HBOT led to significant improvements in physical function, cognitive function, and quality of life in individuals with CFS. Similarly, case reports and anecdotal evidence suggest that HBOT may alleviate symptoms such as fatigue, brain fog, and muscle pain, allowing patients to regain a sense of normalcy and functionality in their daily lives. However, further research is needed to elucidate the mechanisms of action of HBOT in CFS and establish its long-term efficacy and safety in larger, well-controlled clinical trials.

Considerations and Future Directions

While HBOT shows promise as a potential treatment modality for CFS, several considerations must be taken into account in its clinical application. Patient selection, treatment protocols, and outcome measures must be carefully considered to optimize treatment efficacy and safety. Moreover, interdisciplinary collaboration among healthcare providers, researchers, and patients is essential to advance our understanding of CFS and explore new avenues for treatment and management. Future research endeavors should focus on elucidating the underlying pathophysiology of CFS, identifying biomarkers of disease activity and treatment response, and conducting large-scale clinical trials to establish the efficacy and safety of HBOT in this challenging condition. By harnessing the therapeutic potential of HBOT, we may offer new hope and healing to individuals living with the debilitating effects of Chronic Fatigue Syndrome.

Combating Lyme Disease

Lyme disease, caused by the bacterium Borrelia burgdorferi, is a tick-borne illness characterized by a myriad of symptoms, including fatigue, joint pain, neurological impairment, and systemic inflammation. While early detection and treatment with antibiotics can lead to resolution of symptoms in many cases, a subset of individuals may develop persistent or recurrent symptoms, often referred to as chronic Lyme disease or post-treatment Lyme disease syndrome (PTLDS). Hyperbaric Oxygen Therapy (HBOT) has emerged as a potential adjunctive treatment modality for individuals with persistent Lyme disease symptoms, offering new hope for improved outcomes and quality of life.

Pathophysiology of Lyme Disease

Lyme disease is a complex multisystemic illness that can affect various organs and tissues throughout the body. Following a tick bite, the bacterium Borrelia burgdorferi can disseminate via the bloodstream and lymphatic system, leading to systemic infection and inflammatory responses. Early symptoms of Lyme disease may include erythema migrans (bull's-eye rash), flu-like symptoms, and joint pain. If left untreated, Lyme disease can progress to more severe manifestations, including neurological complications (such as meningitis, encephalitis, and peripheral neuropathy), cardiac abnormalities (such as atrioventricular block and myocarditis), and musculoskeletal manifestations (such as arthritis and myositis). While antibiotic therapy is the primary treatment for Lyme disease, a subset of individuals may experience persistent symptoms despite appropriate antibiotic treatment, leading to chronic or recurrent illness.

HBOT holds promise as a potential adjunctive treatment modality for individuals with persistent Lyme disease symptoms due to its ability to enhance tissue oxygenation, modulate inflammatory responses, and potentiate antimicrobial activity. Under hyperbaric conditions, oxygen is dissolved in plasma at supraphysiological levels, promoting oxygen delivery to hypoxic tissues and enhancing cellular metabolism and energy production. This oxygen-rich environment creates unfavorable conditions for bacterial growth and promotes the activity of oxygen-dependent antimicrobial mechanisms, such as oxidative killing by leukocytes and inhibition of microbial metabolism. Moreover, HBOT modulates inflammatory cytokines, such as interleukin-6 (IL-6) and tumor necrosis factor-alpha (TNF-α), reducing neuroinflammation and mitigating symptoms such as fatigue, pain, and cognitive dysfunction associated with Lyme disease.

Clinical Evidence and Outcomes

While clinical research on the use of HBOT in Lyme disease is limited, preliminary studies and case reports suggest that HBOT may offer therapeuticbenefits for individuals with persistent Lyme disease symptoms. For example, a case series by Harch and colleagues (2009) reported improvements in symptoms such as fatigue, cognitive dysfunction, and musculoskeletal pain in patients with chronic Lyme disease who underwent HBOT. Similarly, case reports and anecdotal evidence suggest that HBOT may alleviate symptoms and improve functional outcomes in individuals with persistent Lyme disease symptoms, offering new hope for improved quality of life.

Considerations and Future Directions

Despite the promising potential of HBOT in combating Lyme disease, several considerations must be taken into account in its clinical application. Patient selection, treatment protocols, and outcome measures must be carefully considered to optimize treatment efficacy and safety. Moreover, interdisciplinary collaboration among healthcare providers, researchers, and patients is essential to advance our understanding of Lyme disease and explore new avenues for treatment and management. Future research endeavors should focus on elucidating the underlying pathophysiology of persistent Lyme disease symptoms, identifying biomarkers of disease activity and treatment response, and conducting large-scale clinical trials to establish the efficacy and safety of HBOT in this challenging condition. By harnessing the therapeutic potential of HBOT, we may offer new hope and healing to individuals living with the debilitating effects of chronic Lyme disease.

Supporting Autism Treatment

Autism Spectrum Disorder (ASD) is a neurodevelopmental disorder characterized by deficits in social communication and interaction, restricted interests, repetitive behaviors, and sensory sensitivities. While the etiology of ASD remains poorly understood, emerging evidence suggests that Hyperbaric Oxygen Therapy (HBOT) may offer therapeutic benefits in supporting autism treatment by modulating neuroinflammation, enhancing cerebral blood flow, and improving mitochondrial function.

Challenges in Autism Treatment

Treating autism can be challenging due to the heterogeneity of symptoms and the lack of targeted pharmacological interventions. Behavioral therapies, educational interventions, and supportive services are the mainstays of treatment for individuals with ASD, but these approaches may not address underlying biological abnormalities or provide relief from core symptoms. Moreover, many individuals with ASD experience comorbid medical conditions, such as gastrointestinal issues, immune dysfunction, and mitochondrial dysfunction, which further complicate treatment and management.

HBOT holds promise as a potential adjunctive treatment modality for individuals with ASD due to its ability to modulate neuroinflammation, enhance cerebral blood flow, and improve mitochondrial function. Under hyperbaric conditions, oxygen is dissolved in plasma at supraphysiological levels, promoting oxygen delivery to hypoxic tissues and enhancing cellular metabolism and energy production. This oxygen-rich environment creates favorable conditions for neuronal repair and regeneration, mitigating neuroinflammation and supporting optimal brain function. Moreover, HBOT enhances cerebral blood flow, oxygenation, and glucose metabolism, providing the energy substrates required for neuronal growth and synaptic plasticity. Additionally, HBOT improves mitochondrial function, reduces oxidative stress, and enhances cellular respiration, addressing underlying metabolic abnormalities that may contribute to the pathogenesis of ASD.

Clinical Evidence and Outcomes

While clinical research on the use of HBOT in ASD is still evolving, preliminary studies and case reports suggest that HBOT may offer therapeutic benefits in improving core symptoms and functional outcomes for individuals with ASD. For example, a meta-analysis by Rossignol and colleagues (2012) reported significant improvements in symptoms such as language, social interaction, and sensory sensitivities in children with ASD who underwent HBOT. Similarly, case reports and anecdotal evidence suggest that HBOT may alleviate symptoms and improve quality of life in individuals with ASD, offering new hope for improved outcomes and functionality.

Considerations and Future Directions

Despite the promising potential of HBOT in supporting autism treatment, several considerations must be taken into account in its clinical application. Patient selection, treatment protocols, and outcome measures must be carefully considered to optimize treatment efficacy and safety. Moreover, interdisciplinary collaboration among healthcare providers, researchers, and patients is essential to advance our understanding of ASD and explore new avenues for treatment and management. Future research endeavors should focus on elucidating the underlying pathophysiology of ASD, identifying biomarkers of disease activity and treatment response, and conducting large-scale clinical trials to establish the efficacy and safety of HBOT in this challenging condition. By harnessing the therapeutic potential of HBOT, we may offer new hope and healing to individuals living with the challenges of autism.

Other Emerging Applications

In addition to the established indications discussed above, Hyperbaric Oxygen Therapy (HBOT) is being explored for a myriad of emerging applications across various medical specialties, offering new avenues for healing, recovery, and regeneration. These emerging applications leverage the therapeutic effects of oxygen under increased atmospheric pressure to address a diverse range of conditions, from sports injuries and aesthetic procedures to regenerative medicine and anti-aging interventions.

Sports Medicine and Performance Enhancement

In the realm of sports medicine, HBOT is gaining traction as a potential treatment modality for enhancing recovery from musculoskeletal injuries, reducing inflammation, and improving athletic performance. By promoting tissue oxygenation, angiogenesis, and collagen synthesis, HBOT accelerates the healing of soft tissue injuries, such as muscle strains, ligament sprains, and tendonitis, allowing athletes to return to play more quickly and with reduced risk of complications. Moreover, HBOT reduces oxidative stress, mitigates post-exercise fatigue, and enhances mitochondrial function, providing athletes with the energy required for optimal performance and recovery.

Aesthetic Procedures and Skin Rejuvenation

In aesthetic medicine, HBOT is being explored for its potential to enhance skin rejuvenation, promote collagen synthesis, and improve the outcomes of cosmetic procedures. By increasing tissue oxygenation and promoting fibroblast proliferation, HBOT accelerates wound healing, reduces edema, and enhances skin texture and tone, leading to improved outcomes in procedures such as laser resurfacing, dermal fillers, and chemical peels. Moreover, HBOT stimulates angiogenesis, reduces inflammation, and promotes the production of growth factors, such as vascular endothelial growth factor (VEGF) and transforming growth factor-beta (TGF-β), which play a key role in tissue repair and regeneration.

Regenerative Medicine and Stem Cell Therapy

In regenerative medicine, HBOT holds promise for enhancing the outcomes of stem cell therapy and promoting tissue regeneration in various medical conditions. By creating a hyperoxic environment, HBOT enhances stem cell survival, proliferation, and differentiation, improving their therapeutic efficacy in promoting tissue repair and regeneration. Moreover,

HBOT stimulates angiogenesis, reduces inflammation, and enhances tissue oxygenation, creating favorable conditions for tissue healing and regeneration in conditions such as myocardial infarction, peripheral artery disease, and spinal cord injury.

Anti-Aging Interventions and Longevity

In the realm of anti-aging medicine, HBOT is being explored for its potential to slow the aging process, improve cellular function, and enhance overall health and longevity. By reducing oxidative stress, promoting mitochondrial function, and enhancing cellular metabolism, HBOT combats age-related declines in physiological function and supports optimal cellular health. Moreover, HBOT stimulates the production of growth factors, such as insulin-like growth factor 1 (IGF-1) and brain-derived neurotrophic factor (BDNF), which play a key role in tissue repair, cognitive function, and longevity.

In conclusion, Hyperbaric Oxygen Therapy (HBOT) offers a wealth of emerging applications across various medical specialties, ranging from sports medicine and aesthetic procedures

CHAPTER 4:

Understanding Hyperbaric Chambers

Hyperbaric chambers are essential tools in the delivery of Hyperbaric Oxygen Therapy (HBOT), providing a controlled environment where patients can breathe 100% oxygen at increased atmospheric pressure. In this chapter, we delve into the various types of hyperbaric chambers, their components and operation, as well as the safety measures and regulations governing their use in clinical practice.

Types of Hyperbaric Chambers

Hyperbaric chambers come in different configurations to accommodate the diverse needs of patients and healthcare facilities. The two main categories of hyperbaric chambers are monoplace chambers and multiplace chambers.

Monoplace Chambers:

Monoplace chambers are designed to accommodate a single patient at a time. These chambers are typically cylindrical or tube-like in shape and are pressurized using either pure oxygen or air. Monoplace chambers offer the advantage of providing personalized treatment in a private setting, minimizing the risk of cross-contamination and infection transmission. Additionally, monoplace chambers are often equipped with communication systems and entertainment options to enhance patient comfort during treatment.

Multiplace Chambers:

Multiplace chambers are designed to accommodate multiple patients simultaneously, along with healthcare providers who administer treatment. These chambers are typically larger in size and may resemble a room or compartment with seating arrangements for patients and staff. Multiplace chambers are pressurized using compressed air, and patients breathe 100% oxygen through individual masks or hoods. Multiplace chambers are commonly used in hospital settings where high patient throughput is required, and they facilitate the delivery of HBOT to a larger number of patients in a cost-effective manner.

Components and Operation

Regardless of their type, hyperbaric chambers share common components and operate based on similar principles.

Pressure Vessel:

The pressure vessel is the main structural component of the hyperbaric chamber, designed to withstand high pressures while maintaining a controlled environment for patients. The pressure vessel is constructed from materials such as steel or acrylic and is equipped with viewing windows, access doors, and sealing mechanisms to ensure patient safety and comfort during treatment.

Compression System:

The compression system is responsible for pressurizing the hyperbaric chamber to the desired treatment pressure. In monoplace chambers, compression is achieved using a dedicated compressor that delivers either pure oxygen or compressed air into the chamber. In multiplace chambers, compression is typically achieved using a combination of compressors, valves, and control systems to regulate the flow of compressed air into the chamber.

Oxygen Delivery System:

The oxygen delivery system is responsible for supplying 100% oxygen to patients during HBOT. In monoplace chambers, oxygen is delivered directly to the patient via a breathing hood or mask connected to an oxygen supply system. In multiplace chambers, patients breathe oxygen through individual masks or hoods supplied by a central oxygen distribution system.

Monitoring and Control Systems:

Hyperbaric chambers are equipped with monitoring and control systems to ensure the safety and efficacy of HBOT. These systems include pressure gauges, temperature sensors, oxygen analyzers, and alarms that alert healthcare providers to any deviations from the prescribed treatment parameters. Additionally, modern hyperbaric chambers may be equipped with computerized control systems that allow for precise regulation of pressure, oxygen concentration, and treatment duration.

Safety Measures and Regulations

The use of hyperbaric chambers carries inherent risks, including barotrauma, oxygen toxicity, and fire hazards. To mitigate these risks and ensure patient safety, stringent safety measures and regulations govern the operation of hyperbaric chambers in clinical practice.

Training and Certification:

Healthcare providers who administer HBOT must undergo specialized training and certification to ensure competency in chamber operation, patient assessment, and emergency management. Training programs typically cover topics such as chamber safety protocols, physiological effects of hyperbaric exposure, and emergency procedures.

Patient Screening and Assessment:

Before undergoing HBOT, patients undergo thorough screening and assessment to identify any contraindications or risk factors that may preclude treatment. This includes a comprehensive medical history review, physical examination, and assessment of cardiopulmonary function. Patients with conditions such as untreated pneumothorax, uncontrolled seizures, or recent ear surgery may be deemed ineligible for HBOT due to safety concerns.

Treatment Protocols and Guidelines:

Hyperbaric chambers operate based on standardized treatment protocols and guidelines established by professional organizations such as the Undersea and Hyperbaric Medical Society (UHMS) and the European Committee for Hyperbaric Medicine (ECHM). These guidelines outline recommended indications, treatment parameters, and safety precautions for the use of HBOT in various medical conditions.

Emergency Preparedness:

Hyperbaric facilities must have robust emergency preparedness plans in place to respond to any adverse events or medical emergencies that may arise during HBOT. This includes the availability of emergency medical equipment, such as defibrillators, oxygen resuscitation kits, and airway management devices, as well as trained personnel capable of administering advanced life support interventions.

Regulatory Compliance:

Hyperbaric chambers are subject to regulatory oversight by governmental agencies such as the Food and Drug Administration (FDA) in the United States and the European Medicines Agency (EMA) in Europe. These agencies establish standards for chamber design, construction, and operation, as well as requirements for facility accreditation, personnel training, and quality assurance.

Hyperbaric chambers play a critical role in the delivery of Hyperbaric Oxygen Therapy (HBOT), providing a controlled environment where patients can receive oxygen under increased atmospheric pressure. Understanding the different types of hyperbaric chambers, their components and operation, as well as the safety measures and regulations governing their use, is essential for ensuring the safe and effective delivery of HBOT in clinical practice. By adhering to established guidelines and best practices, healthcare providers can optimize patient outcomes and minimize the risks associated with HBOT, offering new avenues for healing and recovery across a broad spectrum of medical conditions.

CHAPTER 5:

Preparing for Hyperbaric Oxygen Therapy

Preparing for Hyperbaric Oxygen Therapy (HBOT) involves a comprehensive process of patient evaluation, pre-treatment assessments, and education to ensure the safe and effective delivery of therapy. In this chapter, we explore the key considerations and steps involved in preparing patients for HBOT, including patient evaluation and selection, pre-treatment assessments, and patient education and consent.

Patient Evaluation and Selection

Patient evaluation and selection are crucial steps in determining the suitability of individuals for HBOT and optimizing treatment outcomes. Healthcare providers must conduct a thorough assessment of each patient's medical history, current health status, and treatment goals to determine whether HBOT is appropriate and safe for them.

Medical History Review:

Healthcare providers begin by conducting a comprehensive review of the patient's medical history, including past illnesses, surgeries, medications, and allergies. Special attention is paid to conditions that may contraindicate HBOT or increase the risk of complications, such as untreated pneumothorax, uncontrolled seizures, or recent ear surgery.

Physical Examination:

A thorough physical examination is performed to assess the patient's overall health status and identify any signs or symptoms that may impact their ability to tolerate HBOT. This includes assessment of vital signs, cardiopulmonary function, neurological status, and skin integrity.

Diagnostic Testing:

Diagnostic tests may be ordered to further evaluate the patient's medical condition and assess their suitability for HBOT. This may include blood tests, imaging studies (such as X-rays or MRI scans), pulmonary function tests, and audiometric testing. These tests help identify any underlying medical conditions or anatomical abnormalities that may affect the safety or efficacy of HBOT.

Contraindications and Risk Assessment:

Healthcare providers carefully evaluate the patient's medical history, physical examination findings, and diagnostic test results to identify any contraindications or risk factors that may preclude HBOT or increase the risk of complications. Common contraindications to HBOT include untreated pneumothorax, uncontrolled seizures, recent ear surgery, and certain cardiac conditions.

Individualized Treatment Planning:

Based on the patient's medical history, physical examination findings, and diagnostic test results, healthcare providers develop an individualized treatment plan that outlines the recommended course of HBOT, treatment parameters, and goals of therapy. Treatment plans may be adjusted based on the patient's response to therapy and evolving clinical needs.

Pre-Treatment Assessments

Prior to undergoing HBOT, patients undergo a series of pre-treatment assessments to ensure they are adequately prepared for therapy and to minimize the risk of adverse events or complications.

Cardiopulmonary Evaluation

Patients undergo a cardiopulmonary evaluation to assess their cardiovascular and respiratory function and ensure they can tolerate the physiological changes associated with HBOT. This may include assessment of blood pressure, heart rate, oxygen saturation, and lung function tests.

Neurological Assessment:

Patients with neurological conditions or symptoms undergo a neurological assessment to evaluate their cognitive function, sensory perception, and motor function. This helps identify any neurological deficits or impairments that may impact their ability to tolerate HBOT.

Ear, Nose, and Throat Examination:

Patients undergo an ear, nose, and throat examination to assess their auditory and vestibular function and evaluate the integrity of their tympanic membranes. This helps identify any anatomical abnormalities or conditions that may increase the risk of barotrauma or otic complications during HBOT.

Dental Evaluation:

Patients undergo a dental evaluation to assess the health of their teeth and gums and identify any dental issues that may require treatment prior to HBOT. This helps minimize the risk of dental barotrauma or dental complications during therapy.

Psychosocial Assessment:

Patients undergo a psychosocial assessment to evaluate their psychological and emotional well-being and identify any psychosocial factors that may impact their ability to participate in HBOT or adhere to treatment recommendations. This may include assessment of anxiety, depression, coping skills, and social support networks.

Patient Education and Consent

Patient education and consent are essential components of preparing patients for HBOT, providing them with the information and support they need to make informed decisions about their care.

Educational Materials:

Patients receive educational materials that explain the purpose of HBOT, the treatment process, potential benefits and risks, and what to expect during therapy. This may include brochures, pamphlets, videos, and online resources that provide information in a clear and accessible format.

Informed Consent:

Patients provide informed consent before undergoing HBOT, indicating their understanding of the treatment, its potential benefits and risks, and their willingness to participate. Healthcare providers discuss the treatment plan, including alternative options, potential complications, and expected outcomes, and address any questions or concerns the patient may have.

Patient Counseling:

Healthcare providers provide counseling and support to patients throughout the preparation process, addressing any fears, anxieties, or misconceptions they may have about HBOT. This may include discussing coping strategies, relaxation techniques, and ways to manage claustrophobia or anxiety during treatment.

Family Involvement:

Family members or caregivers may be involved in the preparation process, providing support to the patient and assisting with decisionmaking. Healthcare providers may educate family members about the treatment process, potential side effects, and ways they can support the patient before, during, and after HBOT sessions.

Setting Expectations:

It's crucial to set realistic expectations with patients regarding the anticipated outcomes of HBOT. Patients should understand that while HBOT may offer potential benefits for their condition, it may not be a cure-all solution, and results can vary from person to person. Discussing the goals of therapy and the expected timeline for seeing improvement helps manage patient expectations and fosters realistic optimism about the treatment.

Safety Precautions:

Patients are educated about safety precautions to follow before and during HBOT sessions. This includes avoiding smoking and alcohol consumption before treatment, removing all metallic objects and electronic devices, wearing comfortable clothing, and following specific instructions provided by healthcare providers. Patients are also instructed on how to equalize ear pressure during compression and decompression to prevent barotrauma.

Follow-Up Care:

Patients are informed about the importance of follow-up care and monitoring after completing HBOT sessions. They are advised to attend scheduled follow-up appointments with their healthcare provider to assess treatment response, address any concerns or side effects, and make any necessary adjustments to their treatment plan. Patients are encouraged to communicate openly with their healthcare team and report any new symptoms or changes in their condition promptly.

Patient Rights and Responsibilities:

Patients are informed about their rights and responsibilities regarding HBOT treatment. This includes the right to receive respectful and compassionate care, the right to make informed decisions about their treatment, and the responsibility to adhere to treatment recommendations, follow safety protocols, and communicate openly with their healthcare team. Emphasizing patient empowerment and autonomy helps foster a collaborative and therapeutic relationship between patients and providers.

Cultural Sensitivity and Diversity:

Healthcare providers strive to be culturally sensitive and respectful of patients' diverse backgrounds, beliefs, and values. They acknowledge and address any cultural or religious considerations that may impact the patient's experience with HBOT, ensuring that treatment is delivered in a culturally competent and patient-centered manner. This may involve providing educational materials in multiple languages, accommodating cultural preferences regarding modesty or privacy, and engaging interpreters or cultural liaisons as needed.

In conclusion, preparing patients for Hyperbaric Oxygen Therapy (HBOT) involves a multifaceted approach that encompasses patient evaluation and selection, pre-treatment assessments, and patient education and consent. By conducting thorough evaluations, addressing any medical or psychological considerations, and providing patients with the information and support they need to make informed decisions about their care, healthcare providers can ensure the safe and effective delivery of HBOT. Patient education and empowerment are essential components of the preparation process, fostering a collaborative partnership between patients and providers and promoting positive treatment outcomes. By engaging patients as active participants in their care and addressing their individual needs and concerns, healthcare providers can optimize the success of HBOT and help patients achieve their treatment goals.

CHAPTER 6

Hyperbaric Oxygen Therapy Protocols

Hyperbaric Oxygen Therapy (HBOT) protocols outline the standardized procedures and guidelines for the safe and effective delivery of HBOT to patients. In this chapter, we explore the various aspects of HBOT protocols, including standard treatment protocols, adjustments for specific conditions, and monitoring and adjusting treatment plans to optimize patient outcomes.

Standard Treatment Protocols

Standard treatment protocols serve as the foundation for the delivery of HBOT and provide a framework for healthcare providers to follow when administering therapy. These protocols outline the recommended treatment parameters, including treatment pressure, duration, and frequency, as well as safety precautions and monitoring procedures.

Treatment Pressure:

The treatment pressure refers to the level of atmospheric pressure to which the hyperbaric chamber is pressurized during therapy. Standard treatment protocols typically specify a treatment pressure ranging from 2 to 3 atmospheres absolute (ATA), depending on the indication being treated. Higher treatment pressures may be used for conditions such as carbon monoxide poisoning or decompression sickness, while lower pressures may be sufficient for wound healing or adjunctive cancer treatment.

Treatment Duration:

The treatment duration refers to the length of time patients spend inside the hyperbaric chamber during each session. Standard treatment protocols typically recommend treatment durations ranging from 60 to 120 minutes, although this may vary depending on the indication and patient tolerance. Longer treatment durations may be required for conditions such as chronic non-healing wounds, while shorter durations may be sufficient for acute conditions such as carbon monoxide poisoning.

Treatment Frequency:

The treatment frequency refers to the number of HBOT sessions scheduled per week or per month. Standard treatment protocols typically recommend a course of multiple sessions, with sessions scheduled 5 to 7 times per week for acute conditions and 1 to 3 times per week for chronic conditions. The total number of sessions may vary depending on the indication, treatment response, and individual patient factors.

Safety Precautions:

Standard treatment protocols include safety precautions to minimize the risk of adverse events or complications during HBOT. This may include guidelines for patient screening and selection, equipment maintenance and testing, emergency preparedness, and infection control measures. Healthcare providers are trained to follow these protocols rigorously to ensure patient safety and well-being throughout the course of therapy.

Adjustments for Specific Conditions

While standard treatment protocols provide general guidelines for HBOT, adjustments may be necessary to tailor therapy to the specific needs of individual patients and conditions. Healthcare providers must consider factors such as the patient's underlying medical condition, treatment response, and tolerance to therapy when making adjustments to treatment plans.

Contraindications and Cautions:

Certain medical conditions may require adjustments to standard treatment protocols or may be contraindications to HBOT altogether. For example, patients with untreated pneumothorax, uncontrolled seizures, or recent ear surgery may require modifications to treatment parameters or may be ineligible for HBOT due to safety concerns. Healthcare providers carefully evaluate each patient's medical history and condition to determine the appropriateness of therapy and make adjustments as needed.

Treatment Response:

Patients' response to HBOT may vary depending on factors such as the severity of their condition, their overall health status, and individual physiological differences. Healthcare providers monitor patients closely during therapy and adjust treatment parameters based on their response to treatment. This may include modifying treatment pressure, duration, or frequency to optimize therapeutic efficacy and minimize the risk of complications.

Combination Therapies

In some cases, HBOT may be used in combination with other treatment modalities to enhance therapeutic outcomes. Healthcare providers may adjust treatment protocols to accommodate concurrent therapies and ensure compatibility with HBOT. For example, HBOT may be combined with wound care techniques, antibiotic therapy, or surgical interventions to promote wound healing and tissue repair in patients with chronic wounds or infections.

Pediatric and Geriatric Considerations

Special considerations may apply when administering HBOT to pediatric or geriatric patients. Healthcare providers may adjust treatment protocols to account for differences in physiology, metabolism, and tolerance to therapy in these populations. Pediatric patients may require lower treatment pressures or shorter treatment durations to minimize the risk of barotrauma or oxygen toxicity, while geriatric patients may benefit from slower decompression rates or additional monitoring to ensure safety and comfort during therapy.

Monitoring and Adjusting Treatment Plans

Monitoring patients' progress and adjusting treatment plans are integral aspects of HBOT protocols, allowing healthcare providers to optimize therapeutic outcomes and ensure the safety and well-being of patients throughout the course of therapy.

Clinical Assessment:

Healthcare providers conduct regular clinical assessments to monitor patients' progress during HBOT and evaluate their response to treatment. This may include assessing vital signs, symptoms, wound healing progress, and functional status to track improvements over time and identify any changes or complications that may arise during therapy.

Objective Measures:

Objective measures, such as laboratory tests, imaging studies, and physiological assessments, may be used to supplement clinical assessments and provide quantitative data on treatment response. This may include measuring blood oxygen levels, wound healing metrics, cognitive function tests, or radiographic imaging to evaluate changes in disease severity or progression.

Patient Feedback

Patients' feedback and subjective experiences play a crucial role in monitoring treatment response and adjusting therapy as needed. Healthcare providers encourage open communication with patients and solicit feedback on their symptoms, side effects, and overall well-being during HBOT. Patients' input helps guide treatment decisions and ensures that therapy is tailored to their individual needs and preferences.

Collaborative Decision-Making

Treatment plans are developed collaboratively between patients and healthcare providers, taking into account patients' goals, preferences, and treatment priorities. Healthcare providers involve patients in the decision-making process and provide education and support to help them make informed choices about their care. This collaborative approach fosters a sense of partnership and empowerment and ensures that treatment plans align with patients' values and expectations.

Documentation and Record-Keeping

Accurate documentation and record-keeping are essential components of monitoring patients' progress and adjusting treatment plans. Healthcare providers maintain detailed records of each patient's treatment history, including treatment parameters, session dates, clinical assessments, and any adjustments made to treatment plans. This documentation ensures continuity of care, facilitates communication among members of the healthcare team, and provides a comprehensive record of patients' response to therapy.

Interdisciplinary Collaboration

Interdisciplinary collaboration among healthcare providers is critical for monitoring patients' progress and adjusting treatment plans effectively. Healthcare teams may include physicians, nurses, therapists, and other allied health professionals who work together to coordinate care, share information, and make informed decisions about patients' treatment. Regular team meetings, case conferences, and communication channels help ensure that all members of the healthcare team are aligned in their approach to patient care and that treatment plans are adjusted collaboratively based on patients' evolving needs.

Evidence-Based Practice

Healthcare providers rely on evidence-based practice guidelines and clinical research findings to inform their decision-making and adjust treatment plans based on the best available evidence. This may involve reviewing published literature, clinical practice guidelines, and consensus statements from professional organizations to stay abreast of emerging research and best practices in HBOT. By adhering to evidence-based guidelines, healthcare providers can optimize treatment outcomes and ensure that patients receive the most effective and appropriate care.

Patient Education and Empowerment

Throughout the course of HBOT, patients are actively involved in the monitoring process and empowered to participate in decisions regarding their care. Healthcare providers educate patients about the importance of self-monitoring, recognizing signs of treatment response or complications, and communicating openly with their healthcare team. Patients are encouraged to ask questions, express concerns, and provide feedback on their treatment experience, which helps guide adjustments to treatment plans and ensures that therapy remains patient-centered and tailored to individual needs.

Long-Term Follow-Up

After completing HBOT, patients may undergo long-term follow-up to monitor their progress and assess the durability of treatment outcomes. Healthcare providers schedule regular follow-up appointments to evaluate patients' ongoing health status, monitor for any recurrence of symptoms or complications, and make further adjustments to treatment plans as needed. Long-term follow-up helps ensure that patients receive comprehensive care beyond the initial course of therapy and provides opportunities for ongoing support and intervention as required.

Hyperbaric Oxygen Therapy (HBOT) protocols play a critical role in guiding the safe and effective delivery of therapy to patients. Standard treatment protocols provide a framework for healthcare providers to follow, while adjustments for specific conditions, monitoring procedures, and collaborative decision-making help tailor therapy to individual patient needs. By adhering to evidence-based practice guidelines, engaging patients as active participants in their care, and fostering interdisciplinary collaboration among healthcare providers, HBOT protocols can optimize treatment outcomes and ensure that patients receive high-quality, patient-centered care throughout the course of therapy and beyond.

CHAPTER 7:

Clinical Evidence and Research

Hyperbaric Oxygen Therapy (HBOT) has been the subject of numerous clinical studies aimed at evaluating its efficacy, safety, and potential applications across a wide range of medical conditions. In this chapter, we explore the clinical evidence and research surrounding HBOT, including an overview of clinical studies, assessments of efficacy and effectiveness, and areas of ongoing research and debate.

Overview of Clinical Studies

Clinical studies investigating the therapeutic effects of HBOT encompass a diverse array of methodologies, including randomized controlled trials (RCTs), observational studies, case series, and systematic reviews. These studies aim to assess the impact of HBOT on various medical conditions, ranging from wound healing and neurological disorders to radiation injury and carbon monoxide poisoning.

Randomized Controlled Trials (RCTs)

RCTs are considered the gold standard for evaluating the efficacy of medical interventions, including HBOT. In RCTs, participants are randomly assigned to receive either HBOT or a control treatment (e.g., sham treatment or standard care), and outcomes are compared between the two groups. RCTs provide valuable evidence regarding the effectiveness of HBOT and help establish causal relationships between treatment and outcomes.

Observational Studies

Observational studies, such as cohort studies and case-control studies, provide insights into the real-world effectiveness and safety of HBOT in clinical practice. These studies typically involve the collection and analysis of data from patient populations receiving HBOT in routine care settings. While observational studies cannot establish causality like RCTs, they provide valuable information on treatment outcomes, adverse events, and long-term follow-up.

Case Series and Case Reports

Case series and case reports describe the experiences of individual patients or small groups of patients receiving HBOT for specific medical conditions. While these studies offer anecdotal evidence and insights into rare or unusual outcomes, they are considered lower on the hierarchy of evidence and may be subject to biases such as publication bias and selection bias.

Systematic Reviews and Meta-Analyses

Systematic reviews and meta-analyses compile and analyze data from multiple studies to provide a comprehensive summary of the evidence on HBOT for a particular condition. These studies help synthesize the existing literature, identify trends and patterns across studies, and provide quantitative estimates of treatment effects. Systematic reviews and meta-analyses are valuable resources for clinicians, policymakers, and researchers seeking to understand the overall body of evidence on HBOT.

Efficacy and Effectiveness

The efficacy and effectiveness of HBOT have been studied across a wide range of medical conditions, with varying degrees of evidence supporting its use in different contexts. While HBOT has demonstrated efficacy in certain indications, its effectiveness in others remains a subject of ongoing research and debate.

Wound Healing

HBOT is widely recognized as an effective adjunctive treatment for promoting wound healing in various conditions, including diabetic foot ulcers, arterial insufficiency ulcers, and non-healing surgical wounds. Clinical studies have consistently demonstrated improvements in wound healing rates, reduction in wound size, and prevention of amputations in patients receiving HBOT as part of a comprehensive wound care regimen.

Carbon Monoxide Poisoning

HBOT is considered the standard of care for the treatment of carbon monoxide poisoning, as it rapidly eliminates carbon monoxide from the bloodstream and tissues, restores tissue oxygenation, and reduces the risk of long-term neurological sequelae. Randomized controlled trials and observational studies have shown significant reductions in the incidence of neurological deficits and cognitive impairment in patients treated with HBOT for carbon monoxide poisoning.

Decompression Sickness

HBOT is the primary treatment for decompression sickness, a condition that occurs when nitrogen bubbles form in the bloodstream and tissues following rapid decompression, such as during scuba diving. Clinical studies have demonstrated the efficacy of HBOT in promoting bubble resolution, relieving symptoms, and preventing complications in individuals with decompression sickness.

Radiation Injury

HBOT has shown promise as a treatment for radiation-induced tissue injury, such as radiation proctitis, radiation cystitis, and radiation necrosis of the head and neck. While clinical evidence supporting the use of HBOT in these conditions is still evolving, observational studies and case series have reported improvements in symptoms, quality of life, and tissue healing in patients treated with HBOT.

Neurological Disorders

HBOT has been investigated as a potential treatment for various neurological disorders, including traumatic brain injury, stroke, cerebral palsy, and autism spectrum disorder. While some studies have reported positive effects of HBOT on neurological function, cognition, and quality of life in these populations, the evidence remains mixed, and further research is needed to elucidate its role in neurological rehabilitation.

Other Conditions

In addition to the above indications, HBOT has been studied in a wide range of other medical conditions, including inflammatory bowel disease, multiple sclerosis, peripheral arterial disease, and sports-related injuries. While some studies have shown promising results, the overall evidence supporting the use of HBOT in these conditions is limited, and further research is needed to establish its efficacy and effectiveness.

Areas of Ongoing Research and Debate

Despite the wealth of research on HBOT, several areas of ongoing research and debate persist, shaping the future direction of clinical studies and informing clinical practice.

Optimal Treatment Protocols

There is ongoing debate about the optimal treatment protocols for HBOT, including treatment pressure, duration, and frequency. While standard protocols exist for certain indications, such as carbon monoxide poisoning and decompression sickness, the optimal parameters for other conditions remain uncertain and may vary based on patient characteristics and disease severity.

Patient Selection and Predictors of Response

Identifying predictors of response to HBOT and refining patient selection criteria are areas of active research. Factors such as age, comorbidities, disease severity, and genetic predisposition may influence individual responses to HBOT and could help tailor treatment plans to maximize therapeutic efficacy.

Mechanisms of Action

The precise mechanisms underlying the therapeutic effects of HBOT are still not fully understood and continue to be the subject of investigation. While HBOT is known to increase tissue oxygenation, reduce inflammation, and promote tissue repair, the specific cellular and molecular pathways involved remain elusive. Elucidating these mechanisms could lead to the development of novel therapeutic strategies and optimize the use of HBOT in clinical practice.

Combination Therapies

The potential synergistic effects of HBOT in combination with other treatment modalities, such as surgery, antibiotics, and hyperbaric Oxygen Therapy (HBOT) has been the subject of numerous clinical studies aimed at evaluating its efficacy, safety, and potential applications across a wide range of medical conditions. In this chapter, we explore the clinical evidence and research surrounding HBOT, including an overview of clinical studies, assessments of efficacy and effectiveness, and areas of ongoing research and debate.

Overview of Clinical Studies

Clinical studies investigating the therapeutic effects of HBOT encompass a diverse array of methodologies, including randomized controlled trials (RCTs), observational studies, case series, and systematic reviews. These studies aim to assess the impact of HBOT on various medical conditions, ranging from wound healing and neurological disorders to radiation injury and carbon monoxide poisoning.

Randomized Controlled Trials (RCTs)

RCTs are considered the gold standard for evaluating the efficacy of medical interventions, including HBOT. In RCTs, participants are randomly assigned to receive either HBOT or a control treatment (e.g., sham treatment or standard care), and outcomes are compared between the two groups. RCTs provide valuable evidence regarding the effectiveness of HBOT and help establish causal relationships between treatment and outcomes.

Observational Studies

Observational studies, such as cohort studies and case-control studies, provide insights into the real-world effectiveness and safety of HBOT in clinical practice. These studies typically involve the collection and analysis of data from patient populations receiving HBOT in routine care settings. While observational studies cannot establish causality like RCTs, they provide valuable information on treatment outcomes, adverse events, and long-term follow-up.

Case Series and Case Reports

Case series and case reports describe the experiences of individual patients or small groups of patients receiving HBOT for specific medical conditions. While these studies offer anecdotal evidence and insights into rare or unusual outcomes, they are considered lower on the hierarchy of evidence and may be subject to biases such as publication bias and selection bias.

Systematic Reviews and Meta-Analyses

Systematic reviews and meta-analyses compile and analyze data from multiple studies to provide a comprehensive summary of the evidence on HBOT for a particular condition. These studies help synthesize the existing literature, identify trends and patterns across studies, and provide quantitative estimates of treatment effects. Systematic reviews and meta-analyses are valuable resources for clinicians, policymakers, and researchers seeking to understand the overall body of evidence on HBOT.

Efficacy and Effectiveness

The efficacy and effectiveness of HBOT have been studied across a wide range of medical conditions, with varying degrees of evidence supporting its use in different contexts. While HBOT has demonstrated efficacy in certain indications, its effectiveness in others remains a subject of ongoing research and debate.

Wound Healing

HBOT is widely recognized as an effective adjunctive treatment for promoting wound healing in various conditions, including diabetic foot ulcers, arterial insufficiency ulcers, and non-healing surgical wounds. Clinical studies have consistently demonstrated improvements in wound healing rates, reduction in wound size, and prevention of amputations in patients receiving HBOT as part of a comprehensive wound care regimen.

Carbon Monoxide Poisoning

HBOT is considered the standard of care for the treatment of carbon monoxide poisoning, as it rapidly eliminates carbon monoxide from the bloodstream and tissues, restores tissue oxygenation, and reduces the risk of long-term neurological sequelae. Randomized controlled trials and observational studies have shown significant reductions in the incidence of neurological deficits and cognitive impairment in patients treated with HBOT for carbon monoxide poisoning.

Decompression Sickness

HBOT is the primary treatment for decompression sickness, a condition that occurs when nitrogen bubbles form in the bloodstream and tissues following rapid decompression, such as during scuba diving. Clinical studies have demonstrated the efficacy of HBOT in promoting bubble resolution, relieving symptoms, and preventing complications in individuals with decompression sickness.

Radiation Injury

HBOT has shown promise as a treatment for radiation-induced tissue injury, such as radiation proctitis, radiation cystitis, and radiation necrosis of the head and neck. While clinical evidence supporting the use of HBOT in these conditions is still evolving, observational studies and case series have reported improvements in symptoms, quality of life, and tissue healing in patients treated with HBOT.

Neurological Disorders

HBOT has been investigated as a potential treatment for various neurological disorders, including traumatic brain injury, stroke, cerebral palsy, and autism spectrum disorder.

While some studies have reported positive effects of HBOT on neurological function, cognition, and quality of life in these populations, the evidence remains mixed, and further research is needed to elucidate its role in neurological rehabilitation.

In addition to the above indications, HBOT has been studied in a wide range of other medical conditions, including inflammatory bowel disease, multiple sclerosis, peripheral arterial disease, and sports-related injuries. While some studies have shown promising results, the overall evidence supporting the use of HBOT in these conditions is limited, and further research is needed to establish its efficacy and effectiveness.

Despite the wealth of research on HBOT, several areas of ongoing research and debate persist, shaping the future direction of clinical studies and informing clinical practice.

There is ongoing debate about the optimal treatment protocols for HBOT, including treatment pressure, duration, and frequency. While standard protocols exist for certain indications, such as carbon monoxide poisoning and decompression sickness, the optimal parameters for other conditions remain uncertain and may vary based on patient characteristics and disease severity.

Identifying predictors of response to HBOT and refining patient selection criteria are areas of active research. Factors such as age, comorbidities, disease severity, and genetic predisposition may influence individual responses to HBOT and could help tailor treatment plans to maximize therapeutic efficacy.

Mechanisms of Action

The precise mechanisms underlying the therapeutic effects of HBOT are still not fully understood and continue to be the subject of investigation. While HBOT is known to increase tissue oxygenation, reduce inflammation, and promote tissue repair, the specific cellular and molecular pathways involved remain elusive. Elucidating these mechanisms could lead to the development of novel therapeutic strategies and optimize the use of HBOT in clinical practice.

Combination Therapies

The potential synergistic effects of HBOT in combination with other treatment modalities, such as surgery, antibiotics, and hyperbaric adjuncts, are areas of active research. Studies investigating combination therapies aim to identify complementary treatments that enhance the efficacy of HBOT and improve patient outcomes in various medical conditions.

Long-Term Outcomes and Follow-Up

Long-term outcomes and follow-up data are needed to evaluate the durability of treatment effects and assess the impact of HBOT on patient survival, quality of life, and healthcare utilization. Studies with extended follow-up periods provide valuable insights into the long-term benefits and risks of HBOT and help inform decisions regarding its use as a therapeutic intervention.

Cost-Effectiveness and Health Economics:

Assessing the cost-effectiveness and health economic implications of HBOT is an area of growing interest, particularly as healthcare systems face resource constraints and budgetary pressures. Studies evaluating the cost-effectiveness of HBOT compared to standard treatments or alternative interventions help policymakersmake informed decisions about resource allocation and reimbursement policies. Cost-effectiveness analyses consider not only the direct costs associated with HBOT, such as treatment sessions and equipment, but also the indirect costs and potential cost savings associated with improved patient outcomes, reduced hospitalizations, and enhanced quality of life.

Regulatory and Reimbursement Issues

Regulatory oversight and reimbursement policies for HBOT vary across different countries and healthcare systems, contributing to ongoing debates surrounding its accessibility and affordability. Regulatory agencies, such as the U.S. Food and Drug Administration (FDA) and the European Medicines Agency (EMA), play a role in evaluating the safety and effectiveness of HBOT devices and ensuring compliance with quality standards. Reimbursement policies, set by government payers, private insurers, and healthcare providers, determine the extent to which HBOT services are covered and reimbursed, influencing patient access and provider incentives.

Ethical and Legal Considerations

Ethical and legal considerations surrounding HBOT include issues related to patient autonomy, informed consent, medical decision-making, and professional liability. Healthcare providers must ensure that patients are fully informed about the potential risks and benefits of HBOT, as well as any alternative treatment options, so they can make autonomous decisions about their care. Informed consent processes should adhere to ethical principles of respect for patient autonomy, beneficence, non-maleficence, and justice.

Public Perception and Awareness

Public perception and awareness of HBOT influence its acceptance, utilization, and support within communities and healthcare systems. Misconceptions, myths, and controversies surrounding HBOT, fueled by media portrayals and anecdotal reports, can contribute to skepticism and misinformation among patients, providers, and policymakers. Education campaigns, advocacy efforts, and outreach initiatives aimed at increasing public awareness and understanding of HBOT can help dispel myths, clarify misconceptions, and promote evidence-based decision-making.

Global Health Perspectives

Global health perspectives on HBOT encompass considerations of equity, access, and affordability, particularly in low- and middle-income countries where resources may be limited. Disparities in access to HBOT services, driven by socioeconomic factors, geographic location, and healthcare infrastructure, underscore the importance of addressing inequities and ensuring that all patients have access to safe and effective treatments. International collaborations, capacity-building initiatives, and technology transfer programs can help expand access to HBOT and improve health outcomes worldwide.

Future Directions and Emerging Technologies

Future directions for HBOT research and clinical practice include exploring novel applications, refining treatment protocols, and leveraging emerging technologies to enhance therapeutic outcomes. Advances in hyperbaric chamber design, oxygen delivery systems, monitoring technologies, and telemedicine platforms hold promise for improving the safety, efficiency, and accessibility of HBOT services. Multidisciplinary collaborations, translational research efforts, and innovative approaches to patient care are essential for driving continued progress in the field of hyperbaric medicine.

In conclusion, the clinical evidence and research surrounding Hyperbaric Oxygen Therapy (HBOT) encompass a diverse array of studies evaluating its efficacy, safety, and potential applications across various medical conditions. While HBOT has demonstrated effectiveness in certain indications, ongoing research is needed to address areas of uncertainty, refine treatment protocols, and explore novel applications. Debates and controversies surrounding HBOT reflect the complexity of healthcare decision-making, including considerations of evidence, ethics, economics, and equity. By advancing our understanding of HBOT through rigorous research, promoting evidence-based practice, and addressing ethical and regulatory challenges, we can maximize the potential benefits of this therapeutic modality and improve outcomes for patients worldwide.

CHAPTER 8:

Patient Experience and Testimonials

Hyperbaric Oxygen Therapy (HBOT) has impacted the lives of countless individuals, offering hope, healing, and relief from a wide range of medical conditions. In this chapter, we delve into the patient experience and testimonials surrounding HBOT, exploring personal stories of healing and recovery, the challenges and successes faced by patients, and advice for individuals considering or undergoing HBOT treatment.

Personal Stories of Healing and Recovery

The stories of individuals who have undergone HBOT paint a vivid picture of the profound impact this therapy can have on health and well-being. From chronic wounds to neurological disorders, patients across diverse backgrounds and medical histories have shared their journeys of healing and recovery through HBOT.

Wound Healing

For many individuals with chronic wounds, HBOT has been a game-changer, offering new hope and opportunities for healing. Personal stories of individuals with diabetic foot ulcers, venous stasis ulcers, and other non-healing wounds often highlight the transformative effects of HBOT in promoting tissue repair, reducing infection risk, and preventing limb loss. Patients describe how HBOT sessions accelerated wound healing, improved circulation, and restored their quality of life, allowing them to regain mobility and independence.

Neurological Disorders

HBOT has also shown promise in the treatment of various neurological conditions, including traumatic brain injury, stroke, cerebral palsy, and autism spectrum disorder. Personal testimonials from individuals and their caregivers provide insights into the challenges and triumphs of navigating these complex conditions and the role that HBOT has played in their rehabilitation journeys. Patients recount improvements in cognitive function, motor skills, speech, and behavior following HBOT sessions, leading to enhanced communication, independence, and social engagement.

Carbon Monoxide Poisoning and Decompression Sickness

In cases of acute poisoning or injury, HBOT can be life-saving, rapidly eliminating toxins or gases from the bloodstream and tissues. Personal stories from individuals who have experienced carbon monoxide poisoning or decompression sickness underscore the critical importance of timely intervention and access to HBOT services. Survivors share their gratitude for the swift response of healthcare providers and the profound impact that HBOT had on their recovery, preventing long-term neurological damage and enabling them to return to normal activities.

Challenges and Successes

While HBOT offers tremendous potential for healing and recovery, patients may also encounter challenges along the way.

From logistical hurdles to financial concerns, navigating the HBOT journey can be complex and demanding. However, amidst the challenges, patients find moments of triumph and resilience, celebrating the successes and milestones achieved through their perseverance and determination.

Logistical Challenges

One of the primary challenges faced by patients undergoing HBOT is logistical in nature, including scheduling appointments, arranging transportation, and managing treatment logistics. HBOT requires a significant time commitment, with sessions typically lasting 60 to 120 minutes and occurring multiple times per week. Patients may struggle to balance HBOT appointments with work, family obligations, and other healthcare appointments, leading to feelings of stress and overwhelm.

Financial Concerns

Another common challenge for patients undergoing HBOT is the financial burden associated with treatment. While some healthcare providers offer HBOT as a covered service, insurance coverage can vary widely, and out-of-pocket costs may be prohibitive for some patients. Individuals without insurance coverage or access to financial assistance programs may face difficult decisions regarding their ability to pursue HBOT and the potential impact on their finances.

Physical and Emotional Struggles

The physical and emotional toll of living with a chronic illness or injury can be immense, and undergoing HBOT may exacerbate existing symptoms or emotional distress. Patients may experience discomfort or claustrophobia during HBOT sessions, especially in confined spaces such as hyperbaric chambers. Additionally, the uncertainty surrounding treatment outcomes and the fear of the unknown can contribute to feelings of anxiety, depression, or hopelessness.

Family and Caregiver Support

Despite the challenges, patients often find strength and resilience in the support of their families, friends, and caregivers. Personal testimonials frequently highlight the pivotal role that loved ones play in providing emotional support, practical assistance, and encouragement throughout the HBOT journey. Family members and caregivers share in the triumphs and setbacks, celebrating milestones and offering a source of comfort and reassurance during difficult times.

Advice for New Patients

For individuals considering or embarking on the HBOT journey, the insights and advice of those who have walked the path before them can offer valuable guidance and perspective. Patients who have undergone HBOT share their wisdom, lessons learned, and words of encouragement for newcomers navigating the challenges and opportunities of HBOT treatment.

Educate Yourself

One of the most important pieces of advice for new patients is to educate themselves about HBOT and their specific medical condition. Understanding how HBOT works, what to expect during treatment, and the potential benefits and risks can help alleviate anxiety and empower patients to make informed decisions about their care. Patients are encouraged to ask questions, seek information from reliable sources, and engage with their healthcare providers to ensure they have a comprehensive understanding of HBOT and its implications for their health.

Be Patient and Persistent

Healing takes time, and progress may not always be linear. Patients embarking on the HBOT journey are advised to be patient with themselves and their bodies, recognizing that healing is a gradual process that unfolds over time. While setbacks and challenges may arise along the way, perseverance and determination are key. Celebrate small victories, stay focused on the long-term goals, and trust in the healing potential of HBOT.

Build a Support Network

Navigating the HBOT journey can be emotionally and physically demanding, and having a strong support network can make all the difference. New patients are encouraged to lean on their family members, friends, and caregivers for support, encouragement, and practical assistance. Connecting with other individuals who have undergone HBOT or are currently undergoing treatment can also provide valuable insights, camaraderie, and solidarity.

Communicate with Your Healthcare Team

Open and honest communication with healthcare providers is essential for optimizing the HBOT experience and ensuring that patients receive the support and resources they need. New patients are encouraged to communicate their questions, concerns, and treatment preferences with their healthcare team, advocating for their needs and actively participating in decision-making about their care. Healthcare providers serve as partners and guides throughout the HBOT journey, offering expertise, guidance, and compassionate support.

Take Care of Yourself

Self-care is paramount during the HBOT journey, and new patients are reminded to prioritize their physical, emotional, and mental well-being. Engage in activities that promote relaxation, stress reduction, and overall wellness, such as exercise, mindfulness practices, and hobbies. Get plenty of rest, eat a balanced diet, and stay hydrated to support the body's healing process. Remember that self-care is not selfish but essential for sustaining resilience and navigating the challenges of HBOT treatment.

In conclusion, the patient experience and testimonials surrounding Hyperbaric Oxygen Therapy (HBOT) offer a compelling glimpse into the transformative power of this treatment modality. Personal stories of healing and recovery, coupled with insights into the challenges and successes encountered along the way, underscore the profound impact that HBOT can have on individuals' lives. By sharing their experiences, patients offer valuable wisdom and guidance for newcomers embarking on the HBOT

CHAPTER 9:

Integrating Hyperbaric Oxygen Therapy with Other Treatments

Hyperbaric Oxygen Therapy (HBOT) holds promise as a complementary and integrative treatment approach that can be combined with other modalities to enhance patient outcomes. In this chapter, we explore the integration of HBOT with complementary therapies and collaborative approaches in healthcare, highlighting the synergistic benefits of combining treatments to address complex medical conditions.

Complementary Therapies

Complementary therapies encompass a diverse range of healing modalities that can be used alongside conventional medical treatments to promote holistic well-being. When integrated thoughtfully, these therapies can complement the effects of HBOT, addressing not only the physical symptoms of illness but also the emotional, mental, and spiritual dimensions of health.

Nutritional Support

Nutrition plays a crucial role in supporting the body's healing process and optimizing the effectiveness of HBOT. Patients undergoing HBOT may benefit from nutritional counseling and dietary interventions tailored to their specific health needs. A diet rich in antioxidants, vitamins, minerals, and essential nutrients can help enhance cellular repair, boost immune function, and optimize oxygen utilization, complementing the effects of HBOT on tissue healing and recovery.

Physical Therapy

Physical therapy focuses on restoring mobility, strength, and function in individuals with musculoskeletal injuries, neurological disorders, and other conditions. When combined with HBOT, physical therapy can enhance the rehabilitation process, helping patients regain independence, improve balance and coordination, and prevent secondary complications. Integrating physical therapy exercises, stretching routines, and functional movements with HBOT sessions can maximize the benefits of both modalities and accelerate recovery.

Mind-Body Practices

Mind-body practices such as meditation, yoga, tai chi, and mindfulness-based stress reduction techniques offer valuable tools for promoting relaxation, reducing stress, and enhancing overall well-being. When paired with HBOT, these practices can complement the physiological effects of oxygen therapy by promoting a state of calm, reducing inflammation, and supporting mental clarity and resilience. Integrating mind-body practices into the HBOT experience can enhance patient comfort, compliance, and treatment outcomes.

Herbal Medicine and Supplements

Herbal medicine and dietary supplements are commonly used to support health and wellness, offering potential benefits for immune support, inflammation reduction, and tissue repair. While caution should be exercised when combining herbal remedies and supplements with HBOT due to potential interactions and contraindications, judicious use of evidence-based botanicals and nutrients can enhance the therapeutic effects of oxygen therapy and support overall health and vitality.

Acupuncture and Traditional Chinese Medicine

Acupuncture, along with other modalities of Traditional Chinese Medicine (TCM) such as herbal medicine, cupping, and moxibustion, offers a holistic approach to health and healing. When integrated with HBOT, acupuncture can help balance the body's energy meridians, promote circulation, and alleviate pain and inflammation. TCM practitioners may tailor treatment protocols to address specific health concerns and optimize the synergistic effects of acupuncture and HBOT for individual patients.

Collaborative Approaches in Healthcare

Collaborative approaches in healthcare involve coordinated efforts among multidisciplinary teams of healthcare providers to deliver comprehensive, patient-centered care. By working together across different specialties and disciplines, healthcare teams can leverage the unique strengths of each modality to address complex medical conditions more effectively.

Multidisciplinary Care Teams

Multidisciplinary care teams bring together experts from diverse fields, including physicians, nurses, physical therapists, occupational therapists, nutritionists, psychologists, and social workers, to provide comprehensive care for patients undergoing HBOT. Each member of the team contributes their unique expertise and perspective to develop personalized treatment plans, monitor patient progress, and address the complex needs of patients with chronic or acute health conditions.

Care Coordination and Communication

Effective communication and care coordination are essential for ensuring seamless integration of HBOT with other treatments and services. Healthcare providers collaborate closely to share information, coordinate appointments, and monitor patient progress throughout the course of treatment. Regular team meetings, case conferences, and interdisciplinary rounds facilitate communication among team members and ensure that patients receive cohesive, coordinated care across different healthcare settings.

Shared Decision-Making

Shared decision-making involves active collaboration between patients and healthcare providers to make informed decisions about treatment options, based on the best available evidence and patients' preferences, values, and goals. When integrating HBOT with other treatments, healthcare providers engage patients in discussions about their treatment options, potential benefits and risks, and anticipated outcomes, empowering patients to play an active role in their care and treatment decisions.

Evidence-Based Practice

Evidence-based practice involves integrating the best available research evidence with clinical expertise and patient values to inform healthcare decisions and optimize patient outcomes. Healthcare providers rely on evidence-based guidelines, clinical practice protocols, and research findings to guide the integration of HBOT with other treatments, ensuring that interventions are based on sound scientific principles and tailored to individual patient needs and preferences.

Continuous Quality Improvement

Continuous quality improvement involves ongoing evaluation and refinement of healthcare processes and practices to improve patient outcomes, enhance patient safety, and optimize the delivery of care. Healthcare teams involved in the integration of HBOT with other treatments engage in quality improvement initiatives to monitor treatment outcomes, identify areas for improvement, and implement evidence-based interventions to enhance the effectiveness and efficiency of care delivery.

In conclusion, the integration of Hyperbaric Oxygen Therapy (HBOT) with complementary therapies and collaborative approaches in healthcare offers a holistic and patient-centered approach to healing and recovery. By combining the physiological benefits of HBOT with complementary modalities such as nutrition, physical therapy, mind-body practices, and herbal medicine, healthcare providers can address the multifaceted needs of patients and enhance treatment outcomes. Collaborative approaches in healthcare, characterized by multidisciplinary care teams, effective communication, shared decision-making, evidence-based practice, and continuous quality improvement, further optimize the integration of HBOT with other treatments, ensuring that patients receive comprehensive, coordinated, and personalized care. Through thoughtful integration and collaboration, healthcare providers can harness the synergistic benefits of multiple modalities to promote healing, enhance well-being, and improve the overall quality of life for patients undergoing HBOT treatment.

CHAPTER 10

Safety, Risks, and Side Effects

Hyperbaric Oxygen Therapy (HBOT) offers significant therapeutic potential, but like any medical intervention, it comes with its own set of safety considerations, risks, and potential side effects. In this chapter, we delve into the safety aspects of HBOT, exploring common side effects and complications, safety precautions for patients and staff, and regulatory guidelines governing the use of HBOT.

Common Side Effects and Complications

While HBOT is generally considered safe when administered by trained healthcare professionals, certain side effects and complications may occur, particularly in individuals with pre-existing health conditions or risk factors. Understanding these potential adverse effects is essential for ensuring patient safety and well-being during HBOT treatment.

Barotrauma

Barotrauma refers to tissue damage caused by pressure differentials between gas-filled spaces in the body and the surrounding environment. Common forms of barotrauma associated with HBOT include ear barotrauma (e.g., middle ear barotrauma, eustachian tube dysfunction), sinus barotrauma, and dental barotrauma. Patients may experience discomfort, pain, or popping sensations in the ears or sinuses during compression and decompression phases of HBOT. In severe cases, barotrauma can lead to tympanic membrane rupture, sinus barotrauma, or dental injury.

Oxygen Toxicity

Prolonged exposure to high levels of oxygen under hyperbaric conditions can lead to oxygen toxicity, characterized by oxidative stress and tissue damage. Central nervous system oxygen toxicity (CNS-OT) and pulmonary oxygen toxicity (POT) are two main forms of oxygen toxicity associated with HBOT. Symptoms of CNS-OT may include visual disturbances, seizures, nausea, dizziness, and altered mental status. POT can manifest as cough, chest tightness, shortness of breath, and respiratory distress. To mitigate the risk of oxygen toxicity, HBOT protocols typically incorporate intermittent air breaks, limit treatment durations, and monitor oxygen exposure levels closely.

Fire and Explosion Hazard

The use of oxygen-enriched environments in hyperbaric chambers poses a fire and explosion hazard due to the increased flammability of materials in the presence of oxygen. Potential sources of ignition, such as electrical equipment, heating elements, and static electricity, must be carefully controlled to minimize the risk of fire or explosion within the hyperbaric chamber. Fire safety protocols, including the prohibition of flammable materials and the use of explosion-proof equipment, are essential for ensuring the safety of patients and staff during HBOT sessions.

Recompression Chamber

In cases of acute decompression illness, such as decompression sickness or arterial gas embolism, rapid recompression in a hyperbaric chamber is necessary to treat gas bubble formation and restore tissue perfusion. Recompression chamber accidents, while rare, can occur due to equipment malfunction, operator error, or inadequate training. Patients may experience complications such as barotrauma, oxygen toxicity, or exacerbation of existing medical conditions during recompression treatments. Proper training, adherence to safety protocols, and close monitoring of patients are critical to minimizing the risk of adverse events during recompression therapy.

Safety Precautions for Patients and Staff

Ensuring the safety of patients and staff during HBOT sessions requires adherence to strict safety protocols, comprehensive training, and diligent monitoring of treatment parameters. From patient screening to chamber operation, every aspect of HBOT delivery must be carefully managed to minimize risks and maximize safety.

Patient Screening and Evaluation

Before undergoing HBOT, patients undergo a thorough screening and evaluation process to assess their suitability for treatment and identify any contraindications or risk factors. Medical history review, physical examination, and diagnostic testing help healthcare providers determine whether HBOT is appropriate for the patient's condition and whether any precautions or modifications to treatment are necessary.

Chamber Operation and Monitoring

Hyperbaric chambers must be operated and monitored by trained healthcare professionals with expertise in hyperbaric medicine and emergency management. Chamber operators oversee the compression and decompression phases of HBOT, monitor treatment parameters, and respond promptly to any signs of patient distress or equipment malfunction. Continuous monitoring of patient vital signs, oxygen levels, and chamber pressure is essential for ensuring patient safety and well-being throughout the treatment session.

Emergency Preparedness and Response

In the event of a medical emergency or equipment malfunction during HBOT, healthcare providers must be prepared to initiate prompt and effective interventions to ensure patient safety and mitigate risks. Emergency response protocols, including rapid decompression procedures, medical gas administration, and cardiopulmonary resuscitation (CPR), are established to guide healthcare providers in managing emergency situations effectively. Regular training, drills, and simulations help healthcare teams maintain readiness and proficiency in emergency response procedures.

Patient Education and Informed Consent

Patient education and informed consent are essential components of the HBOT treatment process, empowering patients to make informed decisions about their care and treatment options. Healthcare providers educate patients about the potential risks and benefits of HBOT, as well as any alternatives or adjunctive therapies available. Patients are encouraged to ask questions, voice concerns, and actively participate in decision-making about their treatment plan, ensuring that they have a clear understanding of what to expect during HBOT and how to minimize potential risks.

Regulatory Guidelines

Regulatory guidelines govern the safe and effective use of HBOT, outlining standards of practice, quality assurance measures, and safety protocols to protect patients and ensure the integrity of HBOT services.

U.S. Food and Drug Administration (FDA)

The U.S. Food and Drug Administration (FDA) regulates hyperbaric chambers and related medical devices, ensuring their safety, effectiveness, and quality. Hyperbaric chambers intended for medical use must comply with FDA regulations and undergo rigorous testing and evaluation to obtain clearance or approval for marketing. Healthcare facilities offering HBOT services must adhere to FDA regulations governing the operation, maintenance, and safety of hyperbaric chambers, including routine equipment inspections and quality control measures.

Undersea and Hyperbaric Medical Society (UHMS)

The Undersea and Hyperbaric Medical Society (UHMS) establishes clinical practice guidelines, safety standards, and training requirements for healthcare providers practicing hyperbaric medicine. UHMS guidelines cover a wide range of topics, including patient selection criteria, treatment protocols, equipment maintenance, and safety precautions. Healthcare facilities offering HBOT services may voluntarily seek accreditation from the UHMS Hyperbaric Facility Accreditation Program to demonstrate compliance with industry best practices and quality standards.

State and Local Regulations

In addition to federal regulations, state and local governments may impose additional requirements and regulations governing the operation and oversight of HBOT facilities. Licensing requirements, facility inspections, and certification standards may vary by jurisdiction, necessitating compliance with state-specific regulations to ensure legal and ethical practice of hyperbaric medicine.

In conclusion, safety considerations are paramount in the delivery of Hyperbaric Oxygen Therapy (HBOT), requiring careful attention to potential risks, side effects, and safety precautions throughout the treatment process. By understanding common side effects and complications, implementing rigorous safety protocols, and adhering to regulatory guidelines, healthcare providers can ensure the safe and effective delivery of HBOT services while minimizing risks to patients and staff. Through comprehensive patient screening, diligent chamber operation, and emergency preparedness, healthcare teams can create a safe treatment environment that maximizes the therapeutic benefits of HBOT while safeguarding patient well-being. By prioritizing safety, healthcare providers can instill confidence in patients, promote trust in the HBOT

CHAPTER 11:

Future Directions and Innovations

As Hyperbaric Oxygen Therapy (HBOT) continues to evolve, researchers and healthcare professionals are exploring new technologies, applications, and approaches to enhance its effectiveness and expand its therapeutic potential. In this chapter, we explore the future directions and innovations in HBOT, including advances in technology, potential new applications, and the challenges and opportunities that lie ahead.

Advances in Hyperbaric Oxygen Technology

Advances in hyperbaric oxygen technology are driving innovation and improving the safety, efficiency, and accessibility of HBOT. From enhanced chamber designs to innovative oxygen delivery systems, these technological developments are poised to revolutionize the field of hyperbaric medicine.

Next-Generation Hyperbaric Chambers

Next-generation hyperbaric chambers are designed to maximize patient comfort, optimize treatment delivery, and improve safety. Advanced features such as adjustable seating, panoramic views, and integrated entertainment systems enhance the patient experience during HBOT sessions, reducing anxiety and promoting relaxation. Modular chamber designs allow for flexible configuration and scalability, accommodating diverse patient populations and treatment settings. Enhanced safety features, such as redundant systems, automated monitoring, and remote access capabilities, minimize the risk of chamber-related accidents and ensure optimal patient care.

Hyperbaric Oxygen Delivery Systems

Innovations in hyperbaric oxygen delivery systems are transforming the way oxygen is delivered during HBOT sessions, improving oxygenation efficiency and therapeutic outcomes. High-flow oxygen delivery systems, such as hyperbaric oxygen concentrators and membrane oxygenators, offer precise control over oxygen concentration and flow rates, allowing for customized treatment protocols tailored to individual patient needs. Integrated monitoring technologies continuously assess oxygen saturation levels, arterial blood gases, and tissue oxygenation, providing real-time feedback to healthcare providers and optimizing treatment parameters for maximal therapeutic benefit.

Hyperbaric Oxygen Therapy Platforms

Digital health platforms and telemedicine solutions are revolutionizing the delivery of HBOT services, expanding access to care and enhancing patient engagement and outcomes. Telemedicine-enabled hyperbaric chambers allow for remote consultation and supervision by hyperbaric medicine specialists, enabling healthcare providers to deliver expert care and guidance to patients in underserved or remote areas. Integrated health monitoring devices, wearable sensors, and mobile applications facilitate remote patient monitoring, data collection, and treatment optimization, empowering patients to actively participate in their HBOT journey and track their progress over time.

Potential New Applications

The therapeutic potential of HBOT extends beyond its traditional indications, with emerging evidence suggesting novel applications across diverse medical specialties and conditions. From neurodegenerative diseases to chronic inflammatory disorders, researchers are exploring new frontiers in HBOT research and clinical practice.

Neurodegenerative Diseases

HBOT shows promise as a potential therapeutic intervention for neurodegenerative diseases such as

Alzheimer's disease, Parkinson's disease, and amyotrophic lateral sclerosis (ALS). Preclinical studies and early clinical trials have demonstrated neuroprotective effects of HBOT, including reduced neuronal damage, enhanced neurogenesis, and improved cognitive function. Ongoing research is investigating the underlying mechanisms of action and optimal treatment protocols for HBOT in neurodegenerative diseases, with the goal of slowing disease progression and improving quality of life for affected individuals.

Chronic Inflammatory Disorders

Chronic inflammatory disorders, including rheumatoid arthritis, inflammatory bowel disease, and psoriasis, are characterized by dysregulated immune responses and tissue inflammation. HBOT has emerged as a potential adjunctive therapy for these conditions, exerting anti-inflammatory effects, modulating immune function, and promoting tissue repair. Clinical trials and observational studies have demonstrated beneficial effects of HBOT in reducing disease activity, alleviating symptoms, and improving quality of life in patients with chronic inflammatory disorders. Further research is needed to elucidate the underlying mechanisms of action and optimize treatment protocols for HBOT in these conditions.

Sports Performance and Recovery

Athletes and sports enthusiasts are increasingly turning to HBOT as a means of enhancing performance, accelerating recovery, and reducing the risk of sports-related injuries. Hyperbaric training regimens, which involve repeated exposures to hyperbaric oxygen, are thought to stimulate erythropoiesis, increase oxygen delivery to tissues, and enhance aerobic capacity and endurance. HBOT may also promote tissue repair, reduce inflammation, and expedite recovery from sports injuries such as muscle strains, ligament sprains, and stress fractures. While research on the use of HBOT in sports performance and recovery is still limited, anecdotal evidence and preliminary studies suggest potential benefits for athletes seeking a competitive edge.

Challenges and Opportunities

Despite the promise of HBOT, several challenges must be addressed to fully realize its potential and maximize its impact on patient care. From technological barriers to regulatory hurdles, navigating the complexities of HBOT requires collaboration, innovation, and perseverance.

Technological Barriers

Advancing hyperbaric oxygen technology requires overcoming technical challenges related to chamber design, oxygen delivery systems, and monitoring technologies. Engineering solutions that enhance safety, efficiency, and usability of hyperbaric chambers while minimizing costs and resource requirements are needed to expand access to HBOT and facilitate its integration into mainstream healthcare practice.

Regulatory Hurdles

Navigating regulatory frameworks and reimbursement policies for HBOT can be complex and cumbersome, posing barriers to adoption and implementation. Healthcare providers, policymakers, and industry stakeholders must work collaboratively to address regulatory hurdles, streamline approval processes, and advocate for equitable reimbursement policies that ensure patient access to HBOT services.

Research Gaps

While HBOT holds promise for a wide range of medical conditions, gaps in research and evidence remain, hindering its widespread adoption and acceptance within the medical community. Further research is needed to elucidate the underlying mechanisms of action, identify optimal treatment protocols, and evaluate long-term outcomes and cost-effectiveness of HBOT across different patient populations and clinical settings.

Educational Needs

Educating healthcare providers, patients, and the public about the benefits, risks, and appropriate use of HBOT is essential for fostering understanding and acceptance of this therapeutic modality. Continuing medical education programs, clinical practice guidelines, and public awareness campaigns can help bridge knowledge gaps, dispel myths and misconceptions, and promote evidence-based decision-making regarding HBOT.

In conclusion, the future of Hyperbaric Oxygen Therapy (HBOT) is ripe with possibilities, as advances in technology, new applications, and innovative approaches continue to expand its therapeutic potential. By embracing emerging technologies, exploring novel applications, and addressing challenges through collaboration and innovation, healthcare providers can harness the power of HBOT to improve patient outcomes, enhance quality of life, and revolutionize the delivery of healthcare. Through ongoing research, education, and advocacy, we can unlock the full potential of HBOT and pave the way for a future where hyperbaric medicine plays a central role in promoting health and healing for individuals worldwide.

CONCLUSION

In this comprehensive exploration of Hyperbaric Oxygen Therapy (HBOT), we have delved into its history, mechanisms of action, medical applications, technological advancements, safety considerations, and future directions. As we conclude this journey, let us summarize the key points discussed and consider the future of HBOT.

Summary of Key Points

Throughout this book, we have examined the foundations of HBOT, including its historical roots, principles of operation, and mechanisms of action. We have explored its diverse applications across various medical conditions, ranging from wound healing and decompression sickness to neurological disorders and chronic inflammatory conditions. We have also discussed the role of HBOT in enhancing patient outcomes, improving quality of life, and promoting holistic healing.

We have delved into the intricacies of hyperbaric chambers, including their types, components, and operation, as well as safety measures and regulatory guidelines governing their use. We have explored the importance of patient evaluation, pre-treatment assessments, and education in preparing individuals for HBOT and ensuring their safety and well-being throughout the treatment process.

We have examined the standard treatment protocols for HBOT, as well as adjustments for specific conditions and strategies for monitoring and adjusting treatment plans based on patient response. We have explored the clinical evidence and research supporting the efficacy and effectiveness of HBOT, as well as areas of ongoing research and debate in the field.

We have delved into the patient experience and testimonials surrounding HBOT, highlighting personal stories of healing and recovery, as well as the challenges and successes encountered along the way. We have offered advice for new patients embarking on the HBOT journey, emphasizing the importance of education, patience, support, communication, and self-care.

We have explored the integration of HBOT with other treatments, including complementary therapies and collaborative approaches in healthcare, highlighting the synergistic benefits of combining modalities to address complex medical conditions comprehensively. We have discussed safety considerations, risks, and side effects associated with HBOT, as well as safety precautions for patients and staff and regulatory guidelines governing its use.

We have examined future directions and innovations in HBOT, including advances in technology, potential new applications, and the challenges and opportunities that lie ahead. We have considered the role of HBOT in shaping the future of healthcare, promoting health and healing, and improving the quality of life for individuals worldwide.

Looking Ahead

As we look ahead to the future of HBOT, several trends and developments are poised to shape the landscape of hyperbaric medicine in the years to come.

Technological Advancements

Continued advancements in hyperbaric chamber design, oxygen delivery systems, and monitoring technologies will enhance the safety, efficiency, and accessibility of HBOT. Innovations such as next-generation hyperbaric chambers, high-flow oxygen delivery systems, and telemedicine-enabled platforms will expand access to HBOT services and improve patient outcomes.

New Applications and Indications

Emerging research and clinical trials will uncover new applications and indications for HBOT across diverse medical specialties and conditions. From neurodegenerative diseases and chronic inflammatory disorders to sports performance and recovery, HBOT holds promise for addressing unmet medical needs and improving patient care.

Integration and Collaboration

The integration of HBOT with other treatments and collaborative approaches in healthcare will continue to gain traction, as healthcare providers recognize the value of multidisciplinary care and personalized treatment plans. Collaborative efforts among healthcare teams, researchers, policymakers, and industry stakeholders will drive innovation and improve patient outcomes.

Education and Awareness

Educational initiatives and public awareness campaigns will play a crucial role in fostering understanding and acceptance of HBOT among healthcare providers, patients, and the public. By raising awareness of the benefits, risks, and appropriate use of HBOT, we can empower individuals to make informed decisions about their health and explore new avenues for healing and recovery.

In conclusion, Hyperbaric Oxygen Therapy (HBOT) holds tremendous promise as a safe, effective, and versatile treatment modality with the potential to transform healthcare and improve the lives of millions of people worldwide. By embracing technological advancements, exploring new applications, fostering collaboration, and promoting education and awareness, we can unlock the full potential of HBOT and pave the way for a future where hyperbaric medicine plays a central role in promoting health, healing, and well-being for generations to come.

GLOSSARY OF TERMS

Hyperbaric Oxygen Therapy (HBOT) is a complex field with its own set of terminology and jargon. Understanding these terms is essential for healthcare providers, patients, researchers, and anyone interested in the field of hyperbaric medicine. In this glossary, we define and explain key terms related to HBOT, providing clarity and context for their use.

1. Hyperbaric Oxygen Therapy (HBOT)

HBOT is a medical treatment that involves breathing pure oxygen in a pressurized chamber, typically at pressures higher than atmospheric pressure. This increases the partial pressure of oxygen in the bloodstream, allowing oxygen to dissolve more effectively in the plasma and penetrate deeper into tissues, promoting healing and reducing inflammation.

2. Hyperbaric Chamber:

A hyperbaric chamber is a sealed, pressurized enclosure in which HBOT is administered. Hyperbaric chambers come in various designs, including monoplace chambers (for one person) and multiplace chambers (for multiple people). They may be constructed of metal, acrylic, or other materials and are equipped with ventilation systems, communication devices, and monitoring equipment.

3. Barotrauma

Barotrauma refers to tissue damage caused by pressure differentials between gas-filled spaces in the body and the surrounding environment. Common forms of barotrauma associated with HBOT include ear barotrauma (e.g., middle ear barotrauma, eustachian tube dysfunction), sinus barotrauma, and dental barotrauma.

4. Oxygen Toxicity

Oxygen toxicity occurs when the body is exposed to high levels of oxygen for prolonged periods, leading to oxidative stress and tissue damage. Central nervous system oxygen toxicity (CNS-OT) and pulmonary oxygen toxicity (POT) are two main forms of oxygen toxicity associated with HBOT.

5. Decompression Sickness (DCS)

Decompression sickness, also known as "the bends," occurs when dissolved gases (such as nitrogen) form bubbles in the bloodstream and tissues due to rapid decompression. DCS can occur in divers or individuals exposed to changes in atmospheric pressure, leading to symptoms such as joint pain, numbness, tingling, dizziness, and shortness of breath.

6. Carbon Monoxide Poisoning

Carbon monoxide (CO) poisoning occurs when carbon monoxide gas is inhaled, displacing oxygen in the bloodstream and leading to tissue hypoxia. HBOT is used to treat carbon monoxide poisoning by increasing the oxygen content of the blood and accelerating the elimination of carbon monoxide from the body.

7. Wound Healing:

HBOT promotes wound healing by increasing oxygen delivery to injured tissues, stimulating angiogenesis (formation of new blood vessels), enhancing collagen synthesis, and reducing inflammation. It is used to treat chronic non-healing wounds, diabetic foot ulcers, burns, and other types of tissue injuries.

8. Neurological Disorders

HBOT is being investigated as a potential treatment for various neurological disorders, including traumatic brain injury (TBI), stroke, cerebral palsy, multiple sclerosis (MS), and neurodegenerative diseases such as Alzheimer's disease and Parkinson's disease. It may improve oxygenation, reduce inflammation, and promote neuroplasticity in the brain.

9. Pressure

Pressure refers to the force exerted by a gas or fluid on a surface. In the context of HBOT, pressure is typically measured in pounds per square inch absolute (psia) or atmospheres absolute (ATA). The pressure inside a hyperbaric chamber is increased to create a hyperbaric environment conducive to the delivery of oxygen therapy.

10. Treatment Protocol:

A treatment protocol is a set of guidelines or instructions outlining the parameters for administering HBOT to patients. This may include the duration of treatment sessions, the number of treatments prescribed, the pressure levels used, and any specific procedures or precautions to be followed.

11. Contraindication

A contraindication is a specific circumstance or condition in which a particular treatment or intervention is not recommended or should be avoided due to the potential for harm. In the context of HBOT, contraindications may include conditions such as untreated pneumothorax, certain types of lung disease, or certain types of ear or sinus infections.

12. Side Effects:

Side effects are unintended, undesirable effects of a medical treatment or intervention. In the context of HBOT, common side effects may include ear discomfort or pain, sinus pressure, claustrophobia, fatigue, or mild changes in vision. Serious side effects are rare but may include barotrauma, oxygen toxicity, or seizure.

13. Efficacy

Efficacy refers to the ability of a medical treatment or intervention to produce a desired therapeutic effect under controlled conditions. In the context of HBOT, efficacy may be assessed based on clinical outcomes such as wound healing rates, symptom improvement, or disease progression.

14. Safety

Safety refers to the degree to which a medical treatment or intervention poses a risk of harm to patients. In the context of HBOT, safety considerations include the risk of barotrauma, oxygen toxicity, fire or explosion hazard, and potential interactions with other medical conditions or treatments.

15. Regulatory Guidelines

Regulatory guidelines refer to laws, regulations, and standards governing the practice of HBOT, including the operation of hyperbaric chambers, the qualifications of healthcare providers, and the safety and quality of HBOT services. Regulatory agencies such as the U.S. Food and Drug Administration (FDA) and the Undersea and Hyperbaric Medical Society (UHMS) establish guidelines to ensure the safe and effective use of HBOT.

16. Undersea and Hyperbaric Medical Society (UHMS)

The UHMS is a professional medical organization dedicated to promoting research, education, and clinical practice in the fields of undersea and hyperbaric medicine. The UHMS publishes clinical practice guidelines, safety standards, and training requirements for healthcare providers practicing HBOT.

17. Telemedicine

Telemedicine refers to the use of telecommunications technology to provide medical services remotely, allowing patients to consult with healthcare providers and receive care without being physically present in the same location. Telemedicine-enabled hyperbaric chambers allow for remote supervision and consultation by hyperbaric medicine specialists, expanding access to HBOT services in underserved or remote areas.

18. Clinical Evidence

Clinical evidence refers to data derived from clinical trials, observational studies, and other forms of scientific research that support the safety and efficacy of a medical treatment or intervention. In the context of HBOT, clinical evidence may include randomized controlled trials, systematic reviews, meta-analyses, and observational studies evaluating its effects on various medical conditions.

19. Patient Experience

Patient experience refers to the subjective perceptions, feelings, and outcomes reported by patients undergoing HBOT. This may include their level of comfort during treatment, satisfaction with care received, perceived benefits or improvements in symptoms, and overall quality of life. Patient testimonials and anecdotal reports provide valuable insights into the real-world impact of HBOT on individuals' lives.

20. *Integrative Medicine*

Integrative medicine is an approach to healthcare that combines conventional medical treatments with complementary and alternative therapies to address the physical, emotional, and spiritual aspects of health and well-being. HBOT may be integrated into integrative medicine programs alongside other modalities such as acupuncture, massage therapy, nutrition counselling, and stress management techniques.

This glossary provides a comprehensive overview of key terms and concepts related to Hyperbaric Oxygen Therapy (HBOT), offering clarity and understanding for healthcare providers, patients, researchers, and enthusiasts alike. By familiarizing oneself with these terms, individuals can navigate the complexities of HBOT more effectively, communicate with clarity, and make informed decisions about treatment options.

Understanding the terminology surrounding HBOT is crucial for healthcare professionals involved in administering, prescribing, or referring patients for HBOT treatment. Clear communication among interdisciplinary teams ensures the safe and effective delivery of care, facilitates collaboration, and optimizes patient outcomes. Patients, too, benefit from understanding the terminology associated with HBOT, empowering them to engage in meaningful discussions with their healthcare providers, ask informed questions, and actively participate in their treatment journey.

Researchers and scientists studying HBOT rely on precise terminology to accurately describe their findings, communicate results, and contribute to the growing body of evidence supporting the use of HBOT in various medical conditions. By standardizing terminology and definitions, researchers can ensure consistency across studies, facilitate meta-analyses and systematic reviews, and advance our understanding of the mechanisms of action, safety, and efficacy of HBOT.

Furthermore, enthusiasts and advocates for HBOT can use this glossary to deepen their understanding of the field, engage in informed discussions, and advocate for greater access to HBOT services. By raising awareness of the benefits of HBOT and dispelling myths and misconceptions, advocates can promote its integration into mainstream healthcare practice and improve patient access to this valuable therapeutic modality.

As HBOT continues to evolve and expand its reach, maintaining a common understanding of terminology and concepts is essential for fostering collaboration, promoting safety, and advancing the field. By embracing the language of HBOT and staying informed about emerging developments, we can harness the full potential of this innovative therapy to improve health outcomes and enhance quality of life for individuals around the world.

In conclusion, this glossary serves as a valuable resource for anyone interested in HBOT, providing clarity, context, and understanding of the terminology and concepts central to this field. By familiarising themselves with these terms, individuals can navigate the complexities of HBOT more effectively, communicate with clarity, and contribute to the advancement of hyperbaric medicine.